MRCP 1

PASTEST
Dedicated to your success

MRCP 1
Basic Medical Sciences

Best of Five Questions and Answers

Second Edition

Philippa Easterbrook
MB BChir MRCP MPH MD

Professor of HIV Medicine and
Consultant Physician in Infectious Diseases
Guy's, King's and St Thomas' School of Medicine
London

Thushan de Silva
MB ChB Bsc (Hons) DTM&H MRCP

Senior House Officer in HIV Medicine
King's College Hospital
London

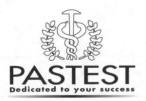

PASTEST
Dedicated to your success

© 2004 PASTEST LTD
Egerton Court
Parkgate Estate
Knutsford
Cheshire
WA16 8DX

Telephone: 01565 752000

First Edition 1996
Second Edition 2004, Reprinted 2006

ISBN: 1 901198 93 6

A catalogue record for this book is available from the British Library.

The information contained within this book was obtained by the authors from reliable sources. However, while every effort has been made to ensure its accuracy, no responsibility for loss, damage or injury occasioned to any person acting or refraining from action as a result of information contained herein can be accepted by the publishers or authors.

PasTest Revision Books and Intensive Courses

PasTest has been established in the field of postgraduate medical education since 1972, providing revision books and intensive study courses for doctors preparing for their professional examinations.

Books and courses are available for the following specialties:
MRCGP, MRCP Parts 1 and 2, MRCPCH Parts 1 and 2, MRCPsych, MRCS, MRCOG Parts 1 and 2, DRCOG, DCH, FRCA, PLAB Parts 1 and 2.

For further details contact:

PasTest, Freepost, Knutsford, Cheshire WA16 7BR
Tel: 01565 752000   Fax: 01565 650264
www.pastest.co.uk   enquiries@pastest.co.uk

Cover design by Parker Design, Northwich, Cheshire
Text prepared by Vision Typesetting Ltd, Manchester
Printed and bound in Europe by the Alden Group

CONTENTS

ACKNOWLEDGEMENT   *page* vii
INTRODUCTION   ix
NORMAL VALUES   xi

1   GENETICS   1
2   MOLECULAR MEDICINE   19
3   MICROBIOLOGY   41
4   IMMUNOLOGY   69
5   ANATOMY   95
6   PHYSIOLOGY   117
7   CLINICAL CHEMISTRY   159
8   STATISTICS AND EPIDEMIOLOGY   185
9   PHARMACOLOGY   201

INDEX   233

Correct answers and teaching notes follow the questions in each chapter.

ACKNOWLEDGEMENT

I wish to thank Mr Kefah Mokbel, currently at St George's Hospital, London, for his contributions to the first edition.

Thanks also to James Greenwood, Specialist Registrar in Respiratory Medicine, Leighton Hospital, Crewe, for his contribution to the Second Edition.

Finally, my thanks go to Cathy Dickens at PasTest for her skill and efficiency during the production of this new edition.

PJE
London 2004

INTRODUCTION

The MRCP Part 1 examination consists of two papers each lasting three hours. Both papers contain 100 'Best of Five' questions (one answer is chosen from five options). The exam is composed of a fixed number of questions drawn from different specialties, which are randomly distributed between both papers. Further details of the exam format are available from www.mrcpuk.org/mrcppt. **A positive marking scheme is used, so that no marks are deducted for a wrong answer.**

One-best Answer/'Best of Five' MCQs

The format of the MRCP Part 1 exam has evolved over a number of years. The purpose of the exam is to test the candidate's ability to apply knowledge and problem-solving skills in the context of a clinical scenario, rather than simply be able to recall isolated facts.

Each 'one-best' MCQ has a question stem, which usually contains clinical information, followed by five branches. All five branches are typically homologous (eg all diagnoses, all laboratory investigations, all antibiotics, etc) and should be set out in a logical order (eg alphabetical). Candidates are asked to select the ONE branch that is the best answer to the question. A response is not required to the other four branches. The answer sheet is, therefore, slightly different to that used for true/false MCQs.

A good strategy that can be used with many well-written one-best MCQs is to try to reach the correct answer without first scrutinising the five options. If you can then find the answer you have reached in the option list, then you are probably correct.

Application of Knowledge and Clinical Problem-solving

A true/false MCQ format had been used in earlier MRCP Part 1 exams, which had been used to test recall of a broad range of factual knowledge. However, the current one-best-answer format is better at testing application of knowledge and problem-solving skills. It is rare that questions included in the exam will have only one possible answer. Most questions will present two or three plausible answers to the stem. Therefore, candidates are assessed on their ability to select the 'best' and most appropriate answer. In order to answer these questions correctly, candidates must *apply* basic knowledge – not just be able to remember it. Unlike the previous true/false MCQ format, there is a much lower chance of randomly guessing the correct stem (20%).

To get the best value from this book you should commit yourself to an answer for each item before you check the correct answer. It is only by being sure of your own responses that you can ascertain which questions you would find difficult in the examination. For each question, an explanation has been provided for why the answer is preferred over the suggested alternatives. However, given the constraints imposed by space, candidates are advised to refer to larger reference texts for more detailed study, and revision texts, for example, *Basic Medical Sciences for MRCP Part 1* by Philippa Easterbrook, published by Elsevier, 2004.

This book contains 318 questions covering Genetics, Molecular Medicine, Immunology, Microbiology, Anatomy, Physiology, Clinical Chemistry, Statistics and Epidemiology, and Clinical Pharmacology. The questions have been updated to reflect recent scientific and clinical developments and presented in the 'best of five' format in accordance with the new MRCP examination requirements. Clinical histories with relevant laboratory and other data have been provided with many questions where appropriate.

PJE
London 2004

NORMAL VALUES

Blood, serum and plasma

Haematology

Haemoglobin	12.5–14.5 g/dl
Mean corpuscular volume (MCV)	80–96 fl
Mean corpuscular haemoglobin (MCH)	28–32 pg
Mean corpuscular haemoglobin concentration (MCHC)	32–35 g/dl
White cell count (WCC)	4–11 × 10^9/l
Differential WCC: neutrophils	1.5–7 × 10^9/l
lymphocytes	1.5–4 × 10^9/l
eosinophils	0.04–0.4 × 10^9/l
Platelet count	150–400 × 10^9/l
Reticulocyte count	50–100 × 10^9/l
Prothrombin time (PT)	12–17 s
Activated partial thromboplastin time (APTT)	24–38 s
Thrombin time (TT)	14–22 s
Fibrinogen	2–5 g/l
Fibrinogen degradation products (FDP)	<10 µg/ml
International normalised ratio (INR)	<1.4
Iron (Fe^{2+})	14–29 µmol/l
Total iron-binding capacity (TIBC)	45–72 µmol/l
Ferritin	15–200 µg/l
Vitamin B$_{12}$	120–700 pmol/l
Folate (serum)	2.0–11.0 µg/l

Red cell folate	160–640 µg/l
Erythrocyte sedimentation rate (ESR)	<12 mm/(1st) hour
Plasma viscosity	1.5–1.72 cP

Immunology/Rheumatology

C-Reactive protein (CRP)	<5mg/l
IgG	6.0–13.0 g/l
IgM	0.4–2.5 g/l
IgA	0.8–3.0 g/l
β_2-Microglobulin	<3 mg/l

Endocrinology

Fasting glucose	3.0–6.0 mmol/l
Hb A_{1c}	3.8–6.4%
Thyroid stimulating hormone (TSH)	0.3–4.0 mU/l
Thyroxine (T4)	58–174 nmol/l
Free T4 (FT4)	10–24 pmol/l
Parathyroid hormone (PTH)	0.8–8.0 pmol/l
Prolactin	<360 mU/l

Biochemistry

Sodium (Na^+)	137–144 mmol/l
Potassium (K^+)	3.5–4.9 mmol/l
Chloride	95–107 mmol/l
Anion gap	12–16 mmol/l
Urea	2.5–7.5 mmol/l
Creatinine	60–110 µmol/l
Calcium (Ca^{2+}), corrected	2.25–2.70 mmol/l
Phosphate	0.8–1.4 mmol/l
Creatine kinase (CK)	<120 U/l
Uric acid	0–0.43 mmol/l
Copper	12–26 µmol/l
Magnesium	0.75–1.05 mmol/l
Lactate	0.6–1.8 mmol/l

Caeruloplasmin	200–350 mg/l
Amylase	60–180 U/l
Plasma osmolality	278–305 mosmol/kg
Alanine aminotransferase (ALT)	5–35 U/l
Aspartate aminotransferase (AST)	1–31 U/l
Alkaline phosphatase (ALP)	20–120 U/l
Lactate dehydrogenase (LDH)	10–250 U/l
Gamma-glutamyl transferase (GGT)	4–35 U/l (<50 U/l in men)
Bilirubin (total)	1–22 µmol/l
Bilirubin (direct, or conjugated)	0–3.4 µmol/l
Total protein	61–76 g/l
Albumin	37–49 g/l
α-Fetoprotein (AFP)	<10–20 µg/l (kU/l)
Cholesterol	<5.2 mmol/l
Triglyceride (fasting)	0.45–1.69 mmol/l

Blood gases

pH	7.36–7.44
PaO_2	11.3–12.6 kPa
$PaCO_2$	4.7–6.0 kPa
Bicarbonate	20–28 mmol/l
Base excess	± 2 mmol/l

Therapeutic drug levels

Digoxin (≥6 h post-dose)	1–2 µg/l
Gentamicin	5–7 µg/ml
Lithium	0.4–1.0 mmol/l

Urine

Albumin	<30 mg/24 h
Albumin/creatinine ratio (random sample)	<2.5 mg/mmol
Total protein	<0.2 g/24 h
Glomerular filtration rate (GFR)	70–140 ml/min
Osmolality	350–1000 mosmol/l

Cerebrospinal fluid (CSF)

Opening pressure	5–18 cmH$_2$O
Total protein	0.15–0.45 g/l
Glucose	3.3–4.4 mmol/l
Cell count	<5 cells/mm^3
Differential cell count: lymphocytes	60–70%
monocytes	30–50%
neutrophils	none

Chapter 1

GENETICS

Questions

1. **Which one of the following conditions has autosomal dominant inheritance?**

   ☐ A Friedreich's ataxia
   ☐ B Haemochromatosis
   ☐ C Agammaglobulinaemia
   ☐ D Malignant hyperthermia
   ☐ E Wilson's disease

2. **Which one of the following statements regarding autosomal recessive inheritance is true?**

   ☐ A If both parents are carriers, then 25% of their children will be carriers
   ☐ B The disease is not usually as severe as a dominantly inherited disease
   ☐ C If one parent is affected and one is not, then 50% of their children will be carriers
   ☐ D It occurs in colour blindness
   ☐ E There is a tendency to skip a generation

3. **Which one of the following disorders is transmitted on the X chromosome?**

   ☐ A Homocystinuria
   ☐ B Phenylketonuria
   ☐ C Marfan's syndrome
   ☐ D Gilbert's syndrome
   ☐ E Glucose-6-phosphate dehydrogenase (G6PD) deficiency

Answers on pages 9–11   1

4. A 25-year-old man suffers from haemophilia, and is troubled with recurrent bleeds into his joints. As a result, he now requires a shoulder replacement. Which one of his relatives may also manifest the disease?

☐ A Father
☐ B Mother
☐ C Sister
☐ D Father's brother
☐ E Mother's brother

5. A 56-year-old woman is diagnosed with primary biliary cirrhosis. She presents to her general practitioner concerned about her condition and wants to know if she is at risk of any other disease processes. Based on her possible HLA typing, which one of the following is she most at risk of developing?

☐ A Myasthenia gravis
☐ B Pernicious anaemia
☐ C Sjögren's syndrome
☐ D Behçet's disease
☐ E Ankylosing spondylitis

6. A 16-year-old boy is known to have cystic fibrosis. This was diagnosed in infancy by means of a sweat test which was performed as part of investigations for failure to thrive. He is quite severely disabled with breathlessness and is admitted to hospital several times a year with severe chest infections. Which one of the following statements about the pattern of inheritance of this disease is true?

☐ A It occurs mainly in males
☐ B Affected individuals usually have an affected parent
☐ C Both parents are homozygous carriers of the gene
☐ D A quarter of the children of two heterozygous parents will be affected
☐ E A quarter of the children of two heterozygous parents will be heterozygous carriers for the trait

7. **Which one of the following statements about DNA structure is correct?**

   ☐ A There are two purine bases called adenine and thymidine
   ☐ B Guanine always pairs with adenine and cytosine with thymidine
   ☐ C An amino acid codon consists of two base pairs
   ☐ D Each strand of DNA has a sugar-phosphate backbone with projecting bases
   ☐ E There are 32 possible codons

8. **Which one of the following chromosomal abnormalities is usually the result of a deletion alone?**

   ☐ A Patau's syndrome
   ☐ B Turner's syndrome
   ☐ C Chronic myeloid leukaemia
   ☐ D Testicular feminisation
   ☐ E Cri-du-chat syndrome

9. **Which one of the following conditions has an autosomal recessive pattern of inheritance?**

   ☐ A Vitamin D-resistant rickets
   ☐ B Cystinuria
   ☐ C Manic depressive illness
   ☐ D Acute intermittent porphyria
   ☐ E Congenital pyloric stenosis

10. **A 19-year-old woman is known to have a 45,XO karyotype. She is short in stature, and inspection reveals a webbed neck and widely spaced nipples. She is of normal intelligence. Which one of the following features may also be associated with this syndrome?**

   ☐ A Tumour of the ovary
   ☐ B Adrenal hyperplasia
   ☐ C Congenital absence of the uterus
   ☐ D Ovarian agenesis
   ☐ E Virilising tumour of the adrenal gland

11. Which one of the following features is characteristically associated with Klinefelter's syndrome?

- ☐ A Increased incidence of breast cancer
- ☐ B Precocious puberty
- ☐ C Coarctation of the aorta
- ☐ D Short metacarpals
- ☐ E Aggressive behaviour

12. Pre-natal testing in a 38-year-old pregnant woman has revealed the presence of Down's syndrome in the fetus. She asks whether individuals with the syndrome are at risk of having other problems with their health. Which one of the following is a feature of Down's syndrome?

- ☐ A Coarctation of the aorta
- ☐ B Primum atrial septal defects
- ☐ C Early development of Alzheimer's disease
- ☐ D Increased prevalence of atherosclerosis
- ☐ E Deletion of chromosome 21

13. Which one of the following is true of Turner's syndrome?

- ☐ A There is an increased risk of neoplasia in the streak ovary
- ☐ B Treatment with growth factor may increase final height
- ☐ C The müllerian structures are absent
- ☐ D There is ambiguity of the external genitalia
- ☐ E Hypertension is rarely seen

14. Which one of the following is true of Charcot–Marie–Tooth disease?

- ☐ A The onset is usually in childhood
- ☐ B There is often mental retardation
- ☐ C It is inherited in an autosomal recessive manner in most cases
- ☐ D Nerve conduction studies may be normal
- ☐ E It only affects the lower limbs

15. Which one of the following is true of the p53 gene (*TP53*)?

A   Its inactivation is often the first event in colorectal carcinoma
B   It is rarely associated with familial breast cancer
C   It is located on chromosome 18q
D   It prevents entry into the S phase of the cell cycle
E   It inhibits apoptosis

16. In a family with hypertrophic obstructive cardiomyopathy (HOCM), which one of the following statements is true?

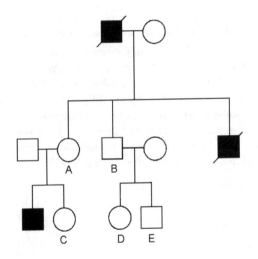

A   The mode of transmission in the family is X-linked recessive inheritance
B   Echocardiography is an essential prerequisite for risk estimation and genetic counselling
C   Approximately 75% of individuals who carry the gene are symptomatic with dyspnoea on exercise and syncope
D   β-Blockers are contraindicated
E   For individuals D and E the risk of inheriting the disease is negligible

Answers on pages 14–15

17. A patient's maternal serum α-fetoprotein (AFP) is found to be elevated above the 97th percentile on a routine antenatal sample at 17 weeks' gestation. Amniocentesis is carried out, which reveals a normal amniotic fluid AFP.Which one of the following is likely to be the cause of the raised maternal AFP?

- [ ] A Open spina bifida
- [ ] B Anterior abdominal wall defect
- [ ] C Congenital nephritic syndrome
- [ ] D Threatened abortion
- [ ] E Fetal skin defects

18. A couple attend the Clinical Genetics Outpatients Clinic for genetic counselling. They both developed emphysematous lung disease at a young age and have mutations consistent with α$_1$-antitrypsin deficiency. He has been a smoker from the age of 18 and began to develop breathlessness around 30 years of age. She has been a life-long non-smoker but began to experience breathlessness at the age of 45. Neither of them has developed liver cirrhosis. What are the chances of their child developing both liver abnormalities and emphysema in childhood?

- [ ] A 10%
- [ ] B 25%
- [ ] C 50%
- [ ] D 75%
- [ ] E 100%

19. Which one of the following statements is true regarding the human genome?

- [ ] A All human cells contain a complete genome
- [ ] B Only 2% of the human genome is composed of genes
- [ ] C Functions are known for approximately 90% of discovered genes
- [ ] D There is a 10% variation in nucleotide bases between people
- [ ] E The human genome consists of around 3 billion genes

20. A 22-year-old Gambian man presents to the Accident and Emergency Department with a two-day history of fevers and rigors. He returned from a three-month trip to The Gambia one week ago. He did not take any antimalarial prophylaxis when he was away as he thought that he was 'immune'. He is unsure, but thinks that there is a history of sickle cell disease in his family. Which one of the following is most true regarding the Hb S allele and *Plasmodium falciparum* malaria?

- [ ] A Heterozygous Hb S disease prevents infection with *P. falciparum*
- [ ] B Homozygous Hb S disease prevents infection with *P. falciparum*
- [ ] C Homozygous Hb S disease prevents death from *P. falciparum* malaria
- [ ] D Infection with *P. falciparum* results in increased sickling of red cells
- [ ] E The frequency of the Hb S allele is increasing in African-Americans

21. A 62-year-old man is seen in the Gastroenterology Outpatients Clinic with a twelve-month history of weight loss and altered bowel habit. A colonoscopy and biopsy has revealed a Dukes' stage B carcinoma in the descending colon. He is concerned that his children might contract the same disease. Which one of the following is true regarding the genetics of this condition?

- [ ] A A single genetic mutation often causes colorectal carcinoma
- [ ] B Approximately 50% of cases are sporadic
- [ ] C The germ-line mutation in the adenomatosis polyposis coli gene (*APC*) is recessively inherited
- [ ] D A mutation in the *APC* gene is seen in 20% of sporadic cases
- [ ] E A deletion in chromosome 18q (the *DCC* gene) is seen in 70% of sporadic cases

22. A 17-year-old girl presents to the Accident and Emergency
     Department with a one-week history of polyuria and polydipsia.
     Her identical twin sister developed type 1 diabetes mellitus at the
     age of 15 years. Both their 72-year-old grandmother and her sister
     are on oral hypoglycaemic medication for type 2 diabetes
     mellitus. Which one of the following is most true regarding the
     inheritance of diabetes mellitus (DM)?

☐ A It usually displays a mendelian pattern of inheritance

☐ B Concordance in monozygotic twins is almost 100% in type 2
       DM

☐ C Concordance in monozygotic twins is approximately 20% in
       type 1 DM

☐ D Risk is independent of the number of first-degree relatives
       affected

☐ E Major histocompatibility complex (MHC) HLA-DR2 is present
       in 98% of cases of type 1 DM and in 50% of cases of type 2
       DM

GENETICS

Answers

1. **D: Malignant hyperthermia**

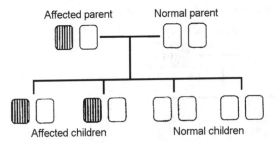

Affected parent   Normal parent

Affected children   Normal children

Autosomal dominant conditions affect both sexes equally. There is no carrier condition, with heterozygotes being phenotypically affected. With one affected parent, 50% of children will be affected.

Autosomal dominant inheritance is seen in:

Achondroplasia
Acute intermittent porphyria
Adult polycystic kidney disease
Ehlers–Danlos syndrome
Familial adenomatous polyposis
Gilbert's syndrome
Hereditary sensory and motor neuropathy
Hereditary spherocytosis
Huntington's disease
Hyperlipidaemia type II
Malignant hyperthermia

Marfan's syndrome
Myotonia congenita
Myotonic dystrophy
Neurofibromatosis
Osteogenesis imperfecta type I
Noonan's syndrome
Polyposis coli
Rotor syndrome
Retinoblastoma
Tuberose sclerosis
Von Hippel–Lindau disease
von Willebrand's disease

2. E: There is a tendency to skip a generation

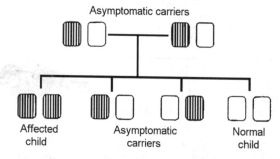

If one parent is affected and one is normal, then all of their children will be carriers. If both parents are carriers, then 50% of their children will be carriers and 25% will be affected. Autosomal recessive disease is usually more severe than autosomal dominant disease. Colour blindness has X-linked inheritance.

The following are **autosomal recessive** conditions:

Albinism
α_1-Antitrypsin deficiency
Ataxia telangectasia
Congenital adrenal hyperplasia
Cystinuria
Cystic fibrosis
Dubin–Johnson syndrome
Familial Mediterranean fever

Fanconi's anaemia
Friedreich's ataxia
Galactosaemia
Gaucher's disease
Glycogen storage diseases
Haemochromatosis
Homocystinuria
Hurler's syndrome
Niemann–Pick disease
Osteogenesis imperfecta types III and IV
Pendred's syndrome
Phenylketonuria
Sickle cell disease
Tay–Sachs disease
Thalassaemias
Wilson's disease

3. **E: Glucose-6-phosphate dehydrogenase (G6PD) deficiency**

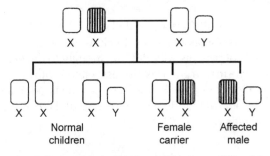

The following are all inherited in an **X-linked** fashion:

Adrenoleukodystrophy
Agammaglobulinaemia
Becker's muscular dystrophy
Chronic granulomatous disease
Colour blindness
Complete testicular feminisation
Duchenne muscular dystrophy
Fabry's disease
Glucose-6-phosphate dehydrogenase deficiency

Haemophilia A (factor VIII deficiency)
Haemophilia B (factor IX deficiency)
Hunter's syndrome
Ichthyosis
Lesch–Nyhan syndromez
Nephrogenic diabetes insipidus
Ocular albinism
Retinitis pigmentosa
Wiskott–Aldrich syndrome

4   E: Mother's brother

Haemophilia is transmitted by female carriers, who produce
affected boys, normal boys, carrier girls and normal girls with equal
frequency. Affected boys and men have affected brothers and
maternal uncles, and can only have normal sons and carrier
daughters. (See answer to Question 3.)

5.   C: Sjögren's syndrome

Primary biliary cirrhosis (PBC) is associated with HLA-DR3.
Sjögren's syndrome is also associated with HLA-DR3 and
approximately 80% of patients with PBC are thought to develop a
sicca syndrome. Myasthenia gravis is also associated with
HLA-DR3 but to a lesser degree. Pernicious anaemia is associated
with HLA-DR2 and HLA-DR5, Behçet's disease with HLA-B5, and
ankylosing spondylitis with HLA-B27.

6.   D: A quarter of the children of two heterozygous parents will be affected

Both sexes are equally affected in disorders with an autosomal
recessive inheritance. Asymptomatic carriers produce affected
children. 'Homozygous' implies that the idividucal is affected.
When both parents carry the gene, one in four children are
affected, and two in four children are carriers. (See answer to
Question 2.)

7. **D: Each strand of DNA has a sugar-phosphate backbone with projecting bases**

The purine bases are adenine (A) and guanine (G); the pyrimidines are thymidine (T) and cytosine (C). G always pairs with C and A with T. An amino acid codon consists of three bases. As each base in the triplet may be any of the four types of nucleotide (A, G, C or T), this results in 64 possible codons. Most amino acids have more than one codon and some codons signal chain termination. Each base in the codon may be one of the four, so there are 4^3 (ie 64) possible codons.

8. **E: Cri-du-chat syndrome**

Approximately 5.6 per 1000 live births are affected by chromosome abnormalities. Of these, 2 per 1000 are caused by a variation in the number of sex chromosomes (Turner's syndrome, 45,XO; Klinefelter's syndrome, 47,XXY); 1.7 per 1000 are due to variation in the number of autosomal chromosomes (Down's syndrome, trisomy 21; Patau's syndrome, trisomy 13; Edwards' syndrome, trisomy 18); and 1.9 per 1000 are due to chromosomal rearrangement. Chronic myeloid leukaemia is associated with the Philadelphia chromosome in 85% of cases: this is a deletion of the long arm of chromosome 22 with translocation, usually onto chromosome 9. Cri-du-chat syndrome is caused by a partial deletion of the short arm of chromosome 5.

9. **B: Cystinuria**

Vitamin D-resistant rickets has X-linked dominant inheritance. Acute intermittent porphyria is an autosomal dominant disorder. Manic depressive illness and congenital pyloric stenosis have polygenic inheritance.

10. **D: Ovarian agenesis**

The phenotypic features of Turner's syndrome (45,XO) comprise a female with short stature, a webbed neck, short metacarpals, a wide carrying angle, sexual infantilism, primary amenorrhoea, high gonadotrophin levels, low oestrogen levels and slight intellectual impairment. Renal abnormalities and coarctation of the aorta are also associated.

11. A: Increased incidence of breast cancer

Klinefelter's syndrome may have a karyotype of 47,XXY, 48,XXYY, 48,XXXY, or 49,XXXXY. The affected male is tall and thin with bilateral gynaecomastia (there is an increased incidence of breast cancer) and infertility (irreversible) due to hypogonadism, and a slight predisposition to germ cell tumours compared with other males. Mental retardation is often seen. Karyotype XYY is usually associated with tall, aggressive men and is commoner in prison communities.

12. C: Early development of Alzheimer's disease

The most common heart defects in Down's syndrome are atrioventricular canal defects (40% compared with 2–3% in the normal population), secundum atrial septal defect and patent ductus arteriosus. Aortic stenosis and coarctation of the aorta are rare. Nearly all people with Down's syndrome have some evidence of Alzheimer's disease by the time they are 40 years old. There is decreased prevalence of atherosclerosis in Down's syndrome, although the reasons for this are not clear. Deletion of chromosome 15q11–q13 is typical of the Prader–Willi syndrome. Trisomy 21 is the classic chromosomal abnormality in Down's syndrome.

13. B: Treatment with growth factor may increase final height

If started sufficiently early enough, large doses of growth hormone may result in increased height. Immature müllerian structures are present. An increased risk of gonadal dysplasia applies only to gonadal dysgenetic syndromes where there is a Y chromosome (eg pure gonadal agenesis, 46,XY). Ambiguity of the external genitalia is not seen. Hypertension is common and is caused by renal abnormalities and coarctation of the aorta.

14. **A: The onset is usually in childhood**

Charcot–Marie–Tooth disease is a hereditary spastic paraparesis which is almost always inherited in an autosomal dominant fashion. The onset is in the first decade, with clinical signs appearing in the legs. The arms may not be affected for years. Nerve conduction velocities are greatly reduced, by definition being less than 30 metres per second.

15. **D: It prevents entry into the S phase of the cell cycle**

The p53 gene is an oncogene found on chromosome 17. Mutations are associated with many common cancers. It is commoner in familial breast cancer syndromes than in sporadic cases. Inactivation of tumour suppressor genes on chromosome 18q is associated with an increased risk of colorectal carcinoma, but inactivation of the p53 pathway is a late event in the majority of colorectal carcinomas. It normally prevents entry into the S phase of the normal cell cycle (DNA replication) until abnormal DNA has been checked and repaired. Other growth-limiting effects include apoptosis and senescence. Screening is possible in affected families.

16. **B: Echocardiography is an essential prerequisite for risk estimation and genetic counselling**

HOCM usually shows an autosomal dominant pattern of transmission. The male-to-male transmission in this family tree rules out an X-linked recessive inheritance. In this condition, expression is very variable and only 25% of carriers of the disease genes are symptomatic. Characteristic echocardiographic abnormalities in those with the HOCM gene include asymmetric ventricular septal hypertrophy, and echocardiography is therefore a prerequisite for genetic counselling. Symptoms may develop at any age and include fatigue, dyspnoea on exercise, angina pectoris and syncope. The prognosis is highly variable, but about 75% of individuals who carry the gene are asymptomatic and have a normal lifespan. Beta-blockers may be effective. Individuals B and C in the diagram have a 1 in 2 chance of inheriting the disease, and for D and E the risk is about 17%.

17. D: Threatened abortion

The causes of elevated maternal serum α-fetoprotein can be divided into two groups:

1. Normal amniotic fluid AFP:
   - normal finding (top 3% of the distribution)
   - wrong dates
   - twins
   - threatened abortion
   - maternal hereditary persistence of AFP
2. Elevated amniotic fluid AFP:
   - encephaly
   - open spina bifida
   - anterior abdominal wall defect
   - congenital nephritic syndrome
   - fetal skin defects.

The test may be offered to any mother who has previously had an affected child. However, about 90% of children born with neural tube defects have mothers with no family history of the disorder. The maternal serum AFP should be repeated and ultrasound examination performed to check the gestational age, to exclude twins, and to look for neural tube defects. If ultrasound examination is normal and a second serum AFP is elevated, amniocentesis is indicated for measurement of amniotic fluid AFP and banding.

18. B: 25%

Alpha$_1$-antitrypsin deficiency is defined by a mutation in the serine (or cysteine) proteinase inhibitor, clade A, member 1 gene (*SERPINA1*) on chromosome 14. It has many different alleles, which produce different amounts of α$_1$-antitrypsin: normal levels (M), moderately low levels (S), very low levels (Z) and none (null). It is inherited in an autosomal recessive fashion and clinical disease is determined by the type and number of alleles inherited. For example, those with a PiZZ phenotype develop childhood emphysema and liver cirrhosis, whereas those with a PiSS phenotype usually produce enough levels to be disease-free. Smoking is an important risk factor in developing emphysema, especially in those with a PiSZ inheritance. Age of onset of emphysema in this group is 32–40 in smokers and 48–54 in non-smokers. Those with a null allele inheritance do not tend to develop liver disease.

In the couple described, the absence of liver cirrhosis and age of onset of their emphysema suggests they both have a PiSZ phenotype (or PiMZ, although this is less likely to cause disease). The chances of their child having a PiZZ phenotype is therefore 25%.

19. **B: Only 2% of the human genome is composed of genes**

The human genome consists of around 3 billion DNA base pairs and approximately thirty to forty thousand genes. All human cells contain a complete genome apart from mature red blood cells. Only 2% of the human genome is composed of genes. The remainder consists of non-coding regions, which may provide structural integrity in chromosomes and regulate where, when and how much of each protein is produced. It has been discovered that 99.9% of nucleotide bases are exactly the same in all people. Currently, functions are unknown for around 50% of discovered genes.

20. **D: Infection with *P. falciparum* results in increased sickling of red cells**

For sickle cell disease in tropical Africa and thalassaemia and G6PD deficiency in the Mediterranean, there is good evidence that a heterozygote state confers an advantage to disease burden with *Plasmodium falciparum*. The genetic resistance is limited to the erythrocytic stage and does not in fact prevent infection from occurring in the first place. In an Hb S heterozygous person, infected red cells show accelerated sickling, which promotes their removal from the circulation. In areas where malaria is endemic homozygotes do not tend to die from cerebral malaria, unlike those with normal red blood cell membranes, but frequently die from causes such as volume depletion, acidosis and cytokine release. It would be expected that the frequency of the Hb S allele is slowly decreasing in areas of reduced exposure to malaria.

21. **E: A deletion in chromosome 18q (the *DCC* gene) is seen in 70% of sporadic cases**

Colorectal carcinogenesis is thought to be a multi-step process, with several mutations present in many sporadic cases. Approximately 70% of all cases are sporadic, fewer than 10% are due to inherited syndromes, and approximately 25% are thought to be familial but with no identified pattern. Both tumour suppressor gene (eg *APC, TP53, DCC*) and oncogene (eg K-*ras*) mutations are implicated in the variety of stages that transform normal colonic mucosa into malignancy. The *APC* gene, when inherited as a germ-line mutation, leads to the autosomal dominant condition, familial adenomatous polyposis (FAP). Somatic mutations of this gene in both alleles are seen in approximately 80% of sporadic cases.

22. **B: Concordance in monozygotic twins is almost 100% in type 2 DM**

Diabetes mellitus (DM) is an example of a multifactorial disorder. These are conditions in which both genetic and environmental factors play a role in development. They follow a 'threshold' model, whereby, despite the presence of contributing genes, the disorder will not manifest until an individual exceeds a certain threshold of liability. Although these disorders tend to recur in families, they do not show mendelian patterns of inheritance. There is 40% concordance for type 1 DM in monozygotic twins and, perhaps surprisingly, almost 100% concordance in monozygotic twins with type 2 DM. Type 1 DM is associated with MHC HLA types DR3, DR4 and B8.

Chapter 2

MOLECULAR MEDICINE

Questions

1. **Which one of the following is true of endothelin?**

☐ A It is a circulating vasoregulatory substance in man
☐ B It has been implicated in the pathogenesis of pulmonary hypertension
☐ C It is raised in the serum of patients with essential hypertension
☐ D It causes bronchodilatation
☐ E Its production is regulated by angiotensin-converting enzyme

2. **A 24-year-old man is admitted to the Intensive Care Unit with severe bilateral pneumonia. Despite being haemodynamically stable, his gas exchange deteriorates and a repeat chest X-ray two days later is consistent with the development of adult respiratory distress syndrome (ARDS). After further increases in positive end-expiratory pressure (PEEP) requirements, he is commenced on inhaled nitric oxide (NO). Which one of the following statements is true regarding endogenous nitric oxide?**

☐ A Synthesis is stimulated by tumour necrosis factor (TNF)
☐ B It acts locally on smooth muscle to cause vasoconstriction
☐ C Its clinical usefulness is increased by its long half-life
☐ D It is a useful treatment for angina
☐ E It directly modulates intracellular processes

Answers on page 27   19

3. **Which one of the following is true of interleukin-1?**

☐ A It cannot be detected in individuals in the absence of inflammation
☐ B Blood levels are a useful index of disease activity in rheumatoid arthritis
☐ C Intravenous infusion leads to hypotension
☐ D It is a neurotransmitter
☐ E It antagonises the effects of TNF

4. **Which one of the following is true of proto-oncogenes?**

☐ A They inactivate oncogenes
☐ B They are carcinogenic retroviruses
☐ C They are down-regulated by growth factors
☐ D They are only expressed in malignant tissues
☐ E They control cell growth

5. **Which one of the following is true of tumour suppressor genes?**

☐ A They are viral in origin
☐ B They exert a dominant effect genetically
☐ C They include the *ras* gene
☐ D They include the *NF-1* gene
☐ E They act to promote cell cycle completion

6. A 21-year-old medical student returns from a two-month elective in Northern India. On arrival in the UK, she develops profuse watery diarrhoea. She is admitted for investigation and intravenous rehydration. Microscopy of her stool reveals curved Gram-negative rods, consistent with *Vibrio cholerae* infection. Which one of the following is true regarding the pathogenesis of *V. cholerae?*

☐ A   G proteins consist of seven main subunits
☐ B   G proteins are activated by the exchange of GDP for GTP
☐ C   Binding of the toxin results in adenylate cyclase down-regulation
☐ D   Cyclic AMP (cAMP) causes reduced cellular chloride secretion
☐ E   Cyclic AMP exerts a negative feedback effect on adenylate cyclase

7. Which one of the following is true of apoptosis?

☐ A   It causes necrotic cell death
☐ B   It is involved in embryonic remodelling
☐ C   It causes an inflammatory reaction
☐ D   It results in an inhibition of phagocytosis
☐ E   It is lost in HIV infection

8. Which one of the following is true of tumour necrosis factor?

☐ A   It is produced by bronchogenic carcinoma
☐ B   It antagonises other inflammatory mediators
☐ C   It is a useful therapy in rheumatoid arthritis
☐ D   Its levels are undetectable in sepsis
☐ E   It causes cachexia

Answers on pages 28–31   21

9. A 21-year-old woman presents to the Clinical Genetics Outpatients Department, concerned about a history of Li–Fraumeni syndrome in her family. Her mother died of multiple associated tumours at the age of 52. The patient has also tested postive for a mutation in the p53 gene (*TP53*). Which one of the following is true of the p53 gene?

    ☐ A   It promotes cell division in adult life
    ☐ B   It is a protein transmitted by viruses
    ☐ C   It is not associated with breast cancer
    ☐ D   It is the commonest genetic mutation in lung cancer
    ☐ E   It is located on chromosome 18q

10. A 27-year-old Asian man presents with a three-week history of headache, confusion, vomiting and photophobia. He lives in a large household, and his uncle has recently been started on antituberculous therapy. You suspect tuberculous meningitis. You perform a lumbar puncture and send a cerebrospinal fluid sample for polymerase chain reaction (PCR) to detect *Mycobacterium tuberculosis*. Which one of the following statements is true of the PCR?

    ☐ A   Only DNA can be used in PCR
    ☐ B   At least 1000 molecules are needed as a template
    ☐ C   The DNA polymerase is stable at room temperature
    ☐ D   DNA strands of up to 1 megabase can be amplified
    ☐ E   No prior knowledge of the template DNA sequence is needed

11. A 32-year-old man with Crohn's disease comes to see you in the clinic. After a clinical assessment which ascertains that he is currently in remission, he asks you about a treatment he has read about on the Internet. He says that treating Crohn's disease with something called 'monoclonal antibodies' has had encouraging results in America, and asks if he would be a candidate for this treatment. Which one of the following is true of monoclonal antibodies?

  A They are derived from human tissue
  B They can be used in medical imaging
  C They are therapeutically useful as they have no side effects
  D They are not in themselves immunogenic
  E They are derived from lymphoma cells

12. Which one of the following is true of cellular signal transduction?

  A It always requires the coupling of G proteins to a second messenger
  B Glucocorticoids bind directly to DNA
  C Second-messenger systems allow amplification of an external stimulus
  D Insulin receptors are ligand-gated ion channels
  E The acetylcholine receptor is a chloride channel

13. With respect to trinucleotide DNA repeats, which one of the following is true?

  A They cause Duchenne muscular dystrophy
  B They result in a later age of onset in successive generations
  C They are unstable in somatic mitosis
  D Huntingdon's disease is caused by a CTG repeat
  E The presence of one repeat usually results in disease

14. **Which one of the following is true of steroid hormone receptors?**

☐ A   They regulate the transcription of certain genes
☐ B   They are functionally similar to most vitamin receptors
☐ C   They have two distinct domains within the cell
☐ D   They act at the same site as peptide hormone receptors
☐ E   They are located on the surface membrane of the cell

15. **Which one of the following is true of interferons?**

☐ A   Interferon-γ and interferon-β act at the same receptors
☐ B   Interferon-γ is a better antiviral agent than interferon-β
☐ C   Interferons are structurally similar to immunoglobulins
☐ D   Interferon-β makes no difference to the MRI appearances of multiple sclerosis
☐ E   Interferon-γ enhances macrophage killing

16. **A 24-year-old intravenous drug user is admitted to hospital with a history of lethargy, fevers and rigors. On examination, a pansystolic murmur is detected and she is commenced on intravenous benzylpenicillin and gentamicin. Over the next few days she develops progressive bilateral sensorineural hearing loss. This is thought to be secondary to ototoxicity caused by gentamicin. Which one of the following statements is true regarding the inheritance of aminoglycoside-induced ototoxicity?**

☐ A   There is poor genotype–phenotype correlation
☐ B   It is transferred by spermatozoa at fertilisation
☐ C   It mutates at a similar rate to nuclear DNA
☐ D   It contains the genes for the enzymes of glycolysis
☐ E   It exhibits homogeneity from cell to cell in the same individual

17. Which one of the following is true of protein synthesis?

- [ ] A It occurs entirely in the nucleus
- [ ] B DNA replication and transcription occurs in a 3′ to 5′ direction
- [ ] C Polypeptide chain formation always starts with methionine
- [ ] D There are two stop codons, UAA and UGA
- [ ] E Translation uses DNA as its template

18. Which one of the following is true of transforming growth factor-β?

- [ ] A It plays a key role in the breakdown of extracellular matrix
- [ ] B It is released from platelets during degranulation
- [ ] C It acts on cell cytosol and nuclear receptors
- [ ] D It promotes the release of proteases
- [ ] E It stimulates lymphocyte proliferation

19. Which one of the following molecule and function pairings is correct?

- [ ] A ras – a guanine nucleotide-binding protein
- [ ] B Integrins – involved in complement-mediated cell lysis
- [ ] C Vitamin B_2 – a principal dietary source of antioxidant
- [ ] D Dystrophin – a form of nerve growth factor
- [ ] E Heat shock proteins – encourage the autodestruction of damaged cells

20. Which one of the following statements about antisense technology is most true?

- [ ] A It involves using modified nucleases to block DNA synthesis
- [ ] B It involves halting the process of DNA transcription to RNA
- [ ] C It relies on endogenous nucleases to aid DNA degradation
- [ ] D It reduces the translation of mRNA into specific proteins
- [ ] E It acts mainly within the nuclear envelope

Answers on pages 35–38

21. **Which one of the following statements is most true of cell senescence?**

   - [ ] A   It is a reversible stage of cell life
   - [ ] B   Metabolic activity is absent
   - [ ] C   There is up-regulation of the p53 gene (*TP53*)
   - [ ] D   There is increased protein turnover
   - [ ] E   Cell division occurs less often

22. **A 25-year-old woman with cystic fibrosis attends her routine Respiratory Outpatients Department appointment. She has had several exacerbations recently which have required hospital admission and is currently on intravenous antibiotics at home. She is worried about her deteriorating condition and is keen to know more about the potential for gene therapy. Which one of the following statements about gene therapy in cystic fibrosis is most true?**

   - [ ] A   It is an example of germ-line gene therapy
   - [ ] B   It involves replacing fragments of DNA within the cystic fibrosis transmembrane conductance regulator gene (*CFTR*)
   - [ ] C   It involves using plasmid DNA as a delivery system
   - [ ] D   It has been attempted using adenoviral vectors
   - [ ] E   It involves the intravenous delivery of a corrected gene

23. **Which one of the following statements about antimicrobials and their site of action is true?**

   - [ ] A   Rifampicin inhibits both prokaryotic and eukaryotic RNA polymerase
   - [ ] B   Trimethoprim inhibits nucleic acid synthesis in prokaryotes only
   - [ ] C   Penicillin and cefuroxime are both inhibitors of DNA gyrase
   - [ ] D   Erythromycin and tetracycline inhibit cell wall synthesis
   - [ ] E   Streptomycin and ciprofloxacin both inhibit protein synthesis

Answers on pages 38–39

MOLECULAR MEDICINE

Answers

1. **B: It has been implicated in the pathogenesis of pulmonary hypertension**

    Endothelins are a family of structurally similar 21-amino acid peptides. Endothelin-1 is the most potent known vasoconstrictor and is produced in the vascular endothelium by the action of endothelin-converting enzyme (ETCE) on pre-proendothelin in response to stress (hypoxia, growth factors, expansion of plasma volume). Endothelins act as paracrine (ie acting on neighbouring cells) regulators of vascular tone and blood pressure, and circulating levels are not relevant to disease processes or to normal homeostasis. Endothelin receptors are found in vascular endothelium and in smooth muscle cells of the lung and gut. It is implicated in the pathogenesis of essential hypertension, primary pulmonary hypertension, chronic cardiac failure, hepatorenal syndrome, Raynaud's phenomenon and vasospasm following subarachnoid haemorrhage. Mutations in the endothelin B receptor are one cause of Hirschsprung's disease and it therefore has a role in the embryonic development of neural crest tissue.

2. **A: Synthesis is stimulated by tumour necrosis factor (TNF)**

    Nitric oxide (NO) is a gas and an important transcellular messenger molecule, which is synthesised from the oxidation of nitrogen atoms in the amino acid L-arginine by the action of NO synthase (NOS). NO acts on target cells close to its site of synthesis where it activates guanylate cyclase, leading to a rise in intracellular cyclic guanosine monophosphate (cGMP) which acts in turn as a second messenger to modulate a variety of cellular processes. It has a very short half-life, and is broken down rapidly in the circulation to nitrates and nitrites. The expression of NO is controlled by the distribution of NOS, which has a constitutive (ie produced at a basal level) isoform active in the brain (mediating memory formation) and in vascular endothelium (causing vasodilatation). It also has an inducible form in mononuclear phagocytes (part of the innate immune response activated by cytokines and involved in the killing of microorganisms). NO is also a free radical which can interact with other reactive oxygen species to lead to lipid peroxidation of cell membranes and subsequent cell death. Synthetic nitrates, such as glyceryl trinitrate and sodium nitroprusside, act after their conversion into NO. NO-mediated processes are implicated in the following clinical situations:

1. Atherosclerosis (where loss of NO-dependent vasodilatation leads to vasospasm)
2. Cell death in the central nervous system
3. Hypotension in septic shock
4. Local vasodilatation in ARDS
5. Pulmonary hypertension.

3.   **C: Intravenous infusion leads to hypotension**

Interleukin-1β has a broad spectrum of both beneficial and harmful biological actions and is a central regulator of the inflammatory response. It is synthesised by activated mononuclear phagocytes and secreted into the circulation, where it is cleaved by interleukin-1β-converting enzyme (ICE). Interleukin-1 (IL-1) is of clinical importance in the following:

1. In septic shock IL-1 acts by increasing the concentration of small mediator molecules, such as platelet activating factor (PAF), prostaglandins and nitric oxide, which are potent vasodilators.
2. IL-1 is present in the synovial lining and fluid of patients with rheumatoid arthritis and it is thought to activate gene expression for collagenases, phospholipases and cyclooxygenases. Serum levels are not relevant to disease activity.

3. IL-1 has some host defence properties, inducing T and B lymphocytes, and reduces mortality from bacterial and fungal infection in animal models.

4. **E: They control cell growth**

   Oncogenes were originally identified as genes carried by cancer-causing viruses. They are the mutated form of normal genes called 'proto-oncogenes' and are usually highly conserved in evolution, with central roles in the signal-transduction pathways that control cell growth and differentiation in eukaryotes. Examples of the range of cellular processes affected are given below:

Classification	Example	Function
Growth factors	*sis*	Platelet-derived growth factor
Growth factor receptors	*trk*	Receptor for nerve growth factor
Intracellular transducers	*ras*	G protein
Nuclear transcription factors	*myc*	DNA-binding protein

   Only one mutated copy of the gene is required to promote malignant growth because, by definition, the mutation of the gene leads to activation. Growth factors transiently up-regulate proto-oncogenes and it is only oncogenes that are virus-related.

5. **A: They are viral in origin**

   Tumour suppressor genes, in contrast to oncogenes, exert a recessive effect in that two 'hits' are required before loss of function and tumorigenesis occur. Several types of inherited cancers involve this mechanism, for example the tumours linked to the *NF-1* gene product 'neurofibromin'. These genes normally function to inhibit the cell cycle and when inactivated lead to loss of growth control. A protein which occupies a pivotal role in the cell cycle is p53, and its gene, *TP53*, is the most commonly mutated gene in tumours (eg breast, colon). It encodes a transcription factor which down-regulates the cell cycle and therefore prevents cells from entering mitosis.

6. **B: G proteins are activated by the exchange of GDP for GTP**

Membrane-bound receptors which are binding sites for an extreme stimulus or first messenger (eg light, hormones, neurotransmitters) interact with second-messenger pathways that are responsible for ultimately leading to a change in the state of the cell surface receptor, leading to initiation of mitosis and cell division. The coupling of first and second messengers via G protein is a ubiquitous and fundamental mechanism in biology. G proteins have three main subunits (α, β, γ). They are attached to GDP under basal conditions, which is exchanged for GTP when a hormone binds. They control many cellular processes, such as neurotransmission, cell division and hormone action. G proteins play a central role in the following disorders:

1. Pseudohypoparathyroidism, where there is generalised resistance to a variety of hormones. The dysmorphic features are caused by a reduction in the activity of the G protein that activates adenylate cyclase in response to hormones such as PTH, T3 and gonadotrophins.
2. In cholera *Vibrio cholerae* secretes an exotoxin that makes a G protein resistant to inactivation and this ultimately leads to fluid and electrolyte loss. Binding of the toxin to the G protein results in activation of adenylate cyclase, which in turn leads to uncontrolled release of intracellular cAMP. There is increased chloride secretion from the cell, as well as reduced sodium absorption from the gut, resulting in watery diarrhoea rich in electrolytes.
3. Mutations activating G proteins occur in about 40% of patients with acromegaly.

7. **B: It is involved in embryonic remodelling**

Apoptosis describes the morphological changes (shrinkage, chromatin condensation and phagocytosis) seen when cells undergo programmed cell death. This is a genetically regulated mechanism for removing unwanted cells, both in embryological development (eg more than 50% of motor neurones die in embryological life) and during adult life, both in health (eg the removal of autoreactive lymphocytes) and disease (eg loss of CD4-positive lymphocytes in AIDS). In contrast to inflammation, apoptosis does not lead to the release of potentially damaging intracellular contents (eg free radicals, proteases) into the surrounding milieu. Cancer can be seen in part as a failure of apoptosis: the oncogene *bcl-2* inhibits cells from entering programmed cell death.

8.   **E: It causes cachexia**

Tumour necrosis factor (TNF) is a pro-inflammatory cytokine released primarily by macrophages in response to inflammatory products, bacterial toxins and other stimuli. The cellular effects of TNF are: cytotoxic damage to tumour cells, reduction of myocyte resting membrane potential, and the suppression of adipocyte lipoprotein lipase. Its effects are similar and complementary to those of IL-1. Overproduction of TNF has been implicated in causing wasting, in mediating septic shock in response to Gram-negative endotoxin, and in autoimmune disorders (anti-TNF antibodies are beneficial in rheumatoid arthritis).

9. D: **It is the commonest genetic mutation in lung cancer**

The p53 protein is coded for by a tumour supressor gene which occupies a pivotal role in the cell cycle and is the most commonly mutated gene in tumours (eg breast, colon, lung). It encodes a transcription factor, whose normal function is to down-regulate the cell cycle by preventing the cells from entering mitosis. This is the primary defect in the Li–Fraumeni syndrome (a familial cancer syndrome involving the development of multiple solid organ tumours) and is a central regulator of apoptosis. Mutation in *TP53* has been associated with lung cancer more often than any other genetic mutation. The gene is located on the 17p chromosome.

10. C: **The DNA polymerase is stable at room temperature**

In the polymerase chain reaction (PCR), DNA which contains a target sequence to be amplified is mixed with oligonucleotide primers (typically 20–30 base pairs in length) and a special heat-stable DNA polymerase derived from a microorganism

(*Thermus aquaticus*) which lives in hot springs. PCR is a way of amplifying a specific region of DNA to produce many copies that can be analysed to detect the presence of specific gene sequences or markers. Its applications in medicine are numerous and include the detection of viral sequences in tissue samples (eg herpes simplex DNA in the CSF in encephalitis) and the diagnosis of specific mutations in genetic diseases and cancer. It is theoretically possible to produce enough DNA by PCR amplification for analysis using only one cell but, in practice, at least 10–100 molecules are needed as a template. RNA can also be used as a template when it has been converted to complementary DNA (cDNA) by reverse transcriptase. With standard techniques the limit of template size that can be amplified is around 2–3 kb.

The Polymerase Chain Reaction

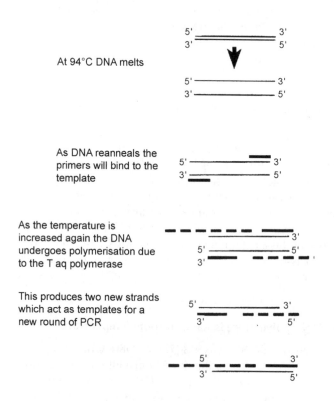

At 94°C DNA melts

As DNA reanneals the primers will bind to the template

As the temperature is increased again the DNA undergoes polymerisation due to the T aq polymerase

This produces two new strands which act as templates for a new round of PCR

11. **B: They can be used in medical imaging**

Monoclonal antibodies are highly specific mouse antibodies which can be produced in large amounts and have found a wide range of applications in medicine. Myeloma is a malignantly transformed B-cell lineage which secretes a specific antibody. This observation is used to produce specific antibodies directed towards an antigen of interest. A laboratory animal, after injection with an antigen of choice, mounts an immune response and its spleen is then harvested. The cells are fused *en masse* to a specialised myeloma cell line which no longer produces its own antibody (this avoids the production of cells which secrete two types of antibody). The resulting fused cells, or hybridomas, constitute an immortalised cell line, and produce antibodies specified by the lymphocytes of the immunised animal. These cells can be screened to select for the antibody of interest which can then be produced in unlimited quantities. Human anti-mouse antibodies (HAMAs) produced by recipients of mouse monoclonals have limited their usefulness. In order to circumvent this problem, monoclonal antibodies can be 'humanised' by joining the antigen-binding site from the mouse antibody to the constant region of human antibodies, thereby retaining specificity while limiting cross-species antigenicity. The clinical applications of monoclonal antibodies include:

1. Diagnosis of cancer and infections
2. Imaging of tumours and radiotherapy
3. Aim to use as a 'magic bullet' to direct anti-rejection drugs
4. In transplantation and other immune modulators.

12. **C: Second-messenger systems allow amplification of an external stimulus**

Although G proteins are a very common way of connecting first messengers to second-messenger systems, this is not the only method used by cells for signal transduction. For example, lipophilic molecules, such as steroids, pass through the cell membrane to interact directly with cytosolic receptors. Many neurotransmitters are the ligand for ion channels, such as the acetylcholine receptor, which is a sodium channel. Some membrane receptors act by direct enzymatic activation of second messengers without the use of G proteins, but most of these systems are characterised by an enormous degree of amplification (ie one first messenger leads ultimately to a cascade of activation of many intracellular molecules).

13.   C: They are unstable in somatic mitosis

Trinucleotide repeats are now recognised to be the cause of a number of genetic neurological diseases. Repeating units of three nucleotides (eg CAG, CTG, CGG) have been found in the coding and non-coding sequences of a number of genes. In most cases there is a variable number of repeats in the general population over a small range: in other words, the number of repeats shows polymorphism. At the upper end of the range the stretch of repeats appears to become unstable during DNA replication and the number of repeats may undergo amplification. If this produces a long enough run of repeats the gene is disrupted and the disease becomes manifest. Because of the unstable nature of trinucleotide repeats, the size of the expansion may increase in successive generations. This provides a molecular explanation for the phenomenon of 'genetic anticipation', in which the offspring of a patient with Huntington's disease, for example, will generally develop the disease earlier and have a larger expansion than their parent. The triplet CTG codes for glutamine and this amino acid has been implicated in so-called 'excitoxic cell death' in the central nervous systm (CNS). It has therefore been proposed that these polyglutamine peptide sequences produced by runs of CTG are in themselves neurotoxic.

Diseases caused by trinucleotide repeats include:

Fragile X mental retardation (CGG)
Friedreich's ataxia (GAA)
Huntington's disease (CAG)
Myotonic dystrophy (CTG)

14. **A: They regulate the transcription of certain genes**

Although all cells contain the same complement of genes (genotype), a nerve cell is clearly different in its morphology and behaviour (phenotype) from a lymphocyte. It is the regulation of gene expression which underlies this difference. Genes are regulated by proteins called 'transcription factors', which bind to specific regions of DNA (located near genes), called 'promoter' and 'enhancer' elements. Transcription factors therefore have specific DNA-binding domains with recurrent structural motifs, which are the basis for their classification. For example, transcription factors with a helix-turn-helix motif are important in developmental regulation in the embryo. The 'zinc finger' motif consists of pairs of amino acids which grasp a zinc atom and push a polypeptide out into a loop (finger) which binds specific regions of DNA.

An example of this kind of transcription factor is the steroid hormone receptor. They are ligand-activated proteins that regulate transcription of certain genes. They have three distinct domains: a ligand-binding domain, a DNA-binding domain and a transcriptional regulatory domain. Steroids act by binding to a receptor, which is part of a complex bound to intracellular cytosolic membrane. When the steroid hormone binds, this releases the hormone receptor complex, which is able to bind to promoter elements on specific genes called 'hormone responsive elements'. Corticosteroids belong to a class of hormones called the 'nuclear hormone superfamily' which all act in this way. This class includes vitamin D, retinoic acid, oestrogens and thyroid hormone.

Transcription factors can act as oncogenes when they are mutated to alter the expression of growth factors. Many hormones and drugs act at the level of transcription factors. Transcription factors may also be a suitable target for gene therapy experiments (eg the up-regulation of fetal haemoglobin in sickle cell anaemia).

15. E: Interferon-γ enhances macrophage killing

Interferon-γ is produced by T lymphocytes and natural killer (NK) cells in response to viral infection. It is an inhibitor of viral replication and mediates a host of other immunological functions, including the up-regulation of MHC class I and II expression and efficiency of macrophage-mediated killing. IFN-γ binds to a specific receptor which is different from that of interferons-α and -β. IFN-γ is an immunomodulator which has been shown to reduce the MRI changes in multiple sclerosis.

16. A: There is poor genotype–phenotype correlation

The tendency to aminoglycoside-induced ototoxicity is inherited via mitochondrial DNA. The mitochondrial genome is circular and approximately 16.5 kb in length. It encodes genes for the mitochondrial respiratory chain and for some species of transfer RNA. No mitochondria are transferred from spermatozoa at fertilisation and so each individual only inherits mtDNA from the mother. Because there are thousands of mitochondria in each cell, the mtDNA content of an individual will be heterogeneous. Mitochondrial DNA mutates ten times more frequently than nuclear DNA. There is poor genotype–phenotype correlation. There is evidence that mtDNA mutations are accumulated throughout life and that this may contribute to the changes of ageing. Several diseases have been shown to be due to mtDNA mutations and these are mostly neurodegenerative diseases with a variable phenotype that can encompass lactic acidosis and diabetes.

17. C: Polypeptide chain formation always starts with methionine

Protein synthesis is a three-stage process involving DNA replication, transcription and translation. The parent DNA is unwound under the control of unwinding proteins, and DNA polymerase synthesises the new strand in a 5' to 3' direction. RNA is made from the DNA template in transcription. This takes place in the nucleus under the control of DNA-dependent RNA polymerase. Translation occurs in the cytoplasm and uses the newly formed mRNA as its template. It always initiates polypeptide chain formation with methionine, and will continue until one of the three stop codons, UAA, UGA or UAG, is reached.

18. **B: It is released from platelets during degranulation**

Transforming growth factor β (TGF-β) is a key cytokine and growth factor that initiates and terminates tissue repair and whose sustained production underlies the development of tissue fibrosis. It acts by binding to specific cell surface receptors which are present on most cell types. The response of a particular cell to TGF-β depends on the presence of other growth factors and the cell type. It has a potent effect on cells to induce the production of extracellular matrix (a dynamic superstructure of self-aggregating macromolecules, including fibronectin, collagen and proteoglycans, which cells attach to by means of surface receptors called 'integrins'). Extracellular matrix is continually being degraded by proteases which are inhibited by TGF-β. It is released by platelets at the site of tissue injury and is strongly chemotactic for monocytes, neutrophils, T cells and fibroblasts. It induces monocytes to begin secreting fibroblast growth factor (FGF), tumour necrosis factor (TNF) and interleukin-1 (IL-1). It also induces its own secretion: this autoinduction may be important in the pathogenesis of fibrosis.

19. **A: ras – a guanine nucleotide-binding protein**

The term 'ras' is an abbreviation for 'rat sarcoma virus' and denotes a family of 21-kDa proteins (H, K and N) found on the cytoplasmic aspect of the plasma membrane. It is a G protein, but of the 'small' monomeric subclass, and is therefore likely to be involved in transduction of growth-promoting signals. At least a third of sporadic tumours contain acquired somatic mutations in the *ras* gene.

Integrins are heterodimeric transmembrane glycoproteins which are widely distributed in different tissues and serve to interact with molecules of the extracellular matrix (eg laminin, fibronectin, collagen).

ANSWERS – MRCP 1 BASIC MEDICAL SCIENCES

Antioxidant molecules are involved in the neutralisation of oxygen-based free radicals which damage cells by lipid peroxidation. The principal dietary sources of antioxidants are vitamins A and C and beta carotene.

Dystrophin is a very large muscle cytoskeleton. Mutations in dystrophin lead to the X-linked progressive muscular dystrophies of Becker and Duchenne.

The 'heat shock response' is a highly conserved and phylogenetically ancient response to tissue stress that is mediated by activation of specific genes. This response leads to an alteration in transcription and the production of specific heat shock proteins that alter the phenotype of the cell. Their diverse functions include the export of proteins in and out of specific cell organelles (acting as molecular 'chaperones'), the catalysis of protein folding and unfolding, and the degradation of proteins (often by the pathway of 'ubiquitination').

20. **D: It reduces the translation of mRNA into specific proteins**

Antisense technology involves using oligonucleotide chemically modified DNA sequences to bind the mRNA of a target gene. This then prevents the translation of the mRNA into a particular protein. It is potentially useful in reducing the expression of particular proteins, for example those implicated in promoting tumour growth. The bcl-2 protein, which has a role in many tumour types, is currently being investigated as a target for antisense technology. Although endogenous nucleases do play a part in destroying the oligonucleotide DNA-mRNA complex, they are proving to be an obstacle to antisense application. Nucleases tend to destroy the drug containing oligonucleotide DNA sequences when it enters the body. The site of action is in the cell cytoplasm, where stable mRNA is found.

21. **C: There is up-regulation of the p53 gene (*TP53*)**

Cell senescence (or 'ageing') is a process that is thought to be important in many diseases of old age, such as Alzheimer's disease.

The cell is no longer capable of dividing, although it is still metabolically active. There is reduced protein turnover and DNA repair. It is generally thought that this is an irreversible stage of cell life and there is up-regulation of the p53 gene, which ultimately leads to an increase in apoptosis. Cell senescence may also be associated with repetitive DNA sequences and the shortening of telomeres, possibly due to the absence of telomerase in somatic cells.

22. D: It has been attempted using adenoviral vectors

Gene therapy for cystic fibrosis is somatic cell therapy, meaning that genetic modifications are targeted specifically at the diseased tissue. Germ-line strategies introduce genetic changes into every cell type. This is currently not allowed and considered unethical, as the changes would be transmitted to future generations. Gene therapy in cystic fibrosis involves insertion of the whole *CFTR* gene, rather than small fragments of DNA to correct specific mutations. Plasmid DNA, although theoretically feasible as a delivery system, does not transfect the respiratory epithelium well enough for practical use. The main methods attempted so far have used viral vectors (retroviruses, adenoviruses) via an aerosol delivery route.

23. B: Trimethoprim inhibits nucleic acid synthesis in prokaryotes only

Rifampicin, streptomycin, tetracycline, chloramphenicol and erythromycin are all inhibitors of prokaryotic protein synthesis. Rifampicin does so by specifically inhibiting prokaryotic RNA polymerase, which in turn blocks the formation of new initiation complexes. Trimethoprim inhibits dihydrofolate reductase in prokaryotes only and thus targets folic acid synthesis (which in turn impairs nucleic acid synthesis). Quinolones, such as ciprofloxacin, inhibit DNA gyrase and prevent DNA from unwinding. Beta-lactam antibiotics prevent cross-link formation in the synthesis of bacterial cell walls.

Chapter 3

MICROBIOLOGY

Questions

1. **An 18-year-old student presents with a two-day history of headache. Now he has vomiting, neck stiffness and photophobia. Lumbar puncture shows Gram-negative diplococci in the cerebrospinal fluid. Which one of the following statements about the likely organism is true?**

   ☐ A It has a polysaccharide capsule
   ☐ B Infection is usually diagnosed by detecting serum antibodies
   ☐ C It is able to survive for long periods outside the human host
   ☐ D It is always pathological in humans
   ☐ E A vaccine is available against all virulent strains

2. **Which one of the following is true of *Listeria monocytogenes*?**

   ☐ A It is a Gram-negative rod
   ☐ B It is usually treated with ciprofloxacin
   ☐ C It can be effectively prevented by vaccination
   ☐ D It can be transmitted through pasteurised milk
   ☐ E It causes meningitis

3. A 60-year-old woman is referred to Casualty by her general practitioner. She has a five-day history of worsening breathlessness, a cough productive of green sputum, and fever. A chest X-ray shows left lower lobe consolidation. Culture of her sputum grows *Haemophilus influenzae*. Which one of the following is true of this organism?

- [ ] A It is a Gram-positive rod
- [ ] B The vaccine is unconjugated
- [ ] C Organisms causing systemic infection are usually encapsulated
- [ ] D It is resistant to amoxicillin
- [ ] E It causes urinary tract infections

4. Infection with which one of these organisms is best treated with penicillin G?

- [ ] A *Escherichia coli*
- [ ] B *Neisseria meningitidis*
- [ ] C *Klebsiella aerogenes*
- [ ] D *Streptococcus faecalis*
- [ ] E *Pseudomonas aeruginosa*

5. Which one of the following virus and disease pairings is correct?

- [ ] A Rotavirus – Lassa fever
- [ ] B Coxsackie B – choroidoretinitis
- [ ] C Flavivirus – yellow fever
- [ ] D HTLV-1 – Ebola virus disease
- [ ] E HTLV-3 – adult T-cell leukaemia

6. While attempting to insert an intravenous cannula into a patient who injects illegal drugs, a preregistration house officer sustains a needlestick injury. The patient mentions that he may have had hepatitis B in the past, and a blood sample is drawn to establish his hepatitis B status. Which one of the following is true of hepatitis B infection?

☐ A   Raised titres of anti-HBs occur during the incubation period of hepatitis B infection

☐ B   The presence of 'e' antigen in serum indicates immunity

☐ C   The risk of transmission with a needlestick injury from a HbsAg-positive source is less than 5%

☐ D   The presence of anti-HBs in the serum indicates immunity

☐ E   Hepatitis B virus is not detectable in the saliva of infected persons

7. Which one of the following is true of HIV infection?

☐ A   Seroconversion following HIV infection generally occurs 3–12 weeks after exposure

☐ B   There is no confirmed association between the acquisition of HIV infection and a history of sexually transmitted disease

☐ C   Disease progression is associated with a fall in the CD4:CD8 ratio and β_2-microglobulin levels

☐ D   Seroconversion following HIV infection is usually asymptomatic

☐ E   The membrane envelope of HIV contains two linked glycoproteins, p24 and p17

8. A patient is referred to you because he is feeling generally unwell
    and has had rigors. He tells you that he has recently returned from
    a holiday in Spain. While he was there, he was moved to a
    different hotel because there was an outbreak of Legionnaires'
    disease. Which one of the following is most true of *Legionella
    pneumophila*?

    ☐   A   It is a Gram-positive coccus
    ☐   B   It causes a rise in cold agglutinin titres
    ☐   C   It is sensitive to erythromycin
    ☐   D   Person-to-person transmission is a potential risk
    ☐   E   It causes haemolytic anaemia

9. A 27-year-old woman who is known to have sickle cell disease
    presents to Casualty with a three-day history of fevers, sweats and
    rigors. Despite opiate analgesia, she continues to complain of
    right thigh pain and a plain X-ray reveals a lesion suspicious of
    osteomyelitis. What is the likely causative organism?

    ☐   A   *Candida albicans*
    ☐   B   *Staphylococcus epidermidis*
    ☐   C   *Staphylococcus aureus*
    ☐   D   *Salmonella* species
    ☐   E   *Streptococcus viridans*

10. Which one of the following statements concerning the congenital
    rubella syndrome is most true?

    ☐   A   Rubella in the third trimester often results in sensorineural
            deafness
    ☐   B   Rubella in the second trimester results in a 90% risk to the baby
    ☐   C   The baby is not infectious after the first week of life
    ☐   D   Ventricular septal defects may occur in the newborn
    ☐   E   Congenital cataracts may be seen in affected neonates

11. **Which one of the following is a contraindication to routine primary vaccination?**

    ☐ A   First trimester of pregnancy
    ☐ B   Age less than six months
    ☐ C   Vaccination during an epidemic
    ☐ D   Infantile eczema
    ☐ E   Previous exposure to disease

12. **Which one of the following features is characteristically associated with congenital toxoplasmosis?**

    ☐ A   The appearance of calcification on the skull X-ray
    ☐ B   The involvement of neonates in successive pregnancies
    ☐ C   Congenital cardiac lesions
    ☐ D   Renal abnormalities
    ☐ E   Congenital cataracts

13. **Over the course of a day in Casualty, you have seen four patients who have all presented with severe abdominal pain, fever, vomiting and diarrhoea. Two of them attended the same wedding a couple of days previously. The microbiologist telephones you the next day to say that their stool samples have grown the O157 strain of *Escherichia coli*. Which one of the following is true of this organism?**

    ☐ A   It bears spores
    ☐ B   It is a non-lactose-fermenter
    ☐ C   It does not grow well anaerobically
    ☐ D   It is a Gram-positive rod
    ☐ E   It is sensitive to vancomycin

14. **Which one of following is most true of Creutzfeldt–Jakob diseases?**

    ☐ A   The majority of cases are familial
    ☐ B   The incubation period is short
    ☐ C   Onset is usually in the second to the fourth decades
    ☐ D   The brain shows demyelination on pathological examination
    ☐ E   There is an equal incidence in men and women

15. Which one of the following infections is a zoonosis?

- ☐ A Trichomoniasis
- ☐ B Tuberculosis
- ☐ C Brucellosis
- ☐ D Amoebiasis
- ☐ E Cholera

16. Exotoxin production is important in the pathogenicity of which one of the following organisms?

- ☐ A *Neisseria meningitidis*
- ☐ B *Klebsiella* species
- ☐ C *Pseudomonas aeruginosa*
- ☐ D *Streptococcus pneumoniae*
- ☐ E *Corynebacterium diphtheriae*

17. A 76-year-old woman who is known to have chronic obstructive pulmonary disease presents with confusion. As part of the infection screen, you send a sputum sample for culture. This is reported as growing 'normal upper respiratory tract flora'. Which one of the following organisms, if present, is likely to be the cause of her disease?

- ☐ A *Neisseria meningitidis*
- ☐ B *Mycobacterium tuberculosis*
- ☐ C *Streptococcus pyogenes*
- ☐ D *Branhamella catarrhalis*
- ☐ E *Haemophilus influenzae* type b

18. Which one of the following conditions is not associated with *Staphylococcus aureus*?

- ☐ A Cholecystitis
- ☐ B Toxic shock syndrome
- ☐ C Acute osteomyelitis
- ☐ D Toxic epidermal necrolysis
- ☐ E Food poisoning

19. **Which one of the following is a characteristic of infection caused by β-lactam-resistant *Staphylococcus aureus*?**

- [ ] A β-Lactam-resistant isolates are less virulent than β-lactam-sensitive strains
- [ ] B Asymptomatic carriage in the nose or rectum of hospital staff is uncommon
- [ ] C Person-to-person transmission is the major route of spread
- [ ] D β-Lactam-resistant strains are sensitive to methicillin
- [ ] E Most strains are coagulase-negative and catalase-positive

20. **A 30-year-old man is known to be HIV-positive. He comes to your clinic as he is planning a trip to Kenya, and wants to know which vaccinations he should have prior to his holiday. Which one of the following vaccines is potentially dangerous in this patient?**

- [ ] A Measles
- [ ] B Hepatitis B
- [ ] C Pneumococcus
- [ ] D BCG
- [ ] E Mumps

21. **Which one of the following is true of the hepatitis C virus?**

- [ ] A It is a DNA virus
- [ ] B It rarely causes chronic liver disease
- [ ] C It may be treated with high-dose aciclovir
- [ ] D It has a prevalence of up to 90% in haemophiliacs
- [ ] E Interferon-β has been shown to improve outcome

22. **Which one of the following statements about *Streptococcus pneumoniae* is true?**

- [ ] A It has five different polysaccharide subtypes
- [ ] B It is an important cause of subacute bacterial endocarditis
- [ ] C It may become resistant to penicillin due to β-lactamase production
- [ ] D It rarely causes infection in people with sickle cell disease
- [ ] E The standard vaccine is rarely effective in children under the age of six years

23. **Which one of the following is true of parvovirus B19?**

☐ A   It is a common cause of diarrhoea in children
☐ B   It is an RNA virus
☐ C   Infection is frequently symptomatic
☐ D   It causes erythema infectiosum
☐ E   It causes persistent anaemia in healthy adults

24. **A 45-year-old woman is referred to the Gastroenterology Department for investigation of reflux-type symptoms. Her mother died of carcinoma of the stomach. Upper gastrointestinal endoscopy shows mild gastritis only. Biopsies taken show *Helicobacter*-like organisms, and the bedside CLO test (for '*Campylobacter*-like organisms') is positive. Which one of the following is true regarding this lady's infection?**

☐ A   The causative organism is found in the mucus which lines the gastric epithelium
☐ B   The causative organism is Gram-positive
☐ C   It is present in 30% of patients with duodenal ulcers
☐ D   Positive serum antibodies indicates continuing infection
☐ E   Repeated antimicrobial courses are usually needed

25. **A diabetic patient presents with pain in his right leg and fever. Examination shows a small ulcer on his right foot, with cellulitis tracking up his leg. A swab of the ulcer reveals a heavy growth of penicillinase-producing staphylococci. To which one of the following antibiotics would this infection be resistant?**

☐ A   Clindamycin
☐ B   Phenoxymethylpenicillin
☐ C   Cefuroxime
☐ D   Ciprofloxacin
☐ E   Vancomycin

26. Which one of the following is true of *Enterococcus faecalis*?

☐ A   It is highly sensitive to penicillin
☐ B   It is associated with food poisoning
☐ C   It may cause haemolysis
☐ D   It is an abnormal finding in healthy individuals
☐ E   It may cause infective endocarditis

27. A 24-year-old woman has just returned from backpacking around India. Since her return she has been suffering from abdominal cramps and profuse watery diarrhoea. On examination she is pale and dehydrated and has a generally tender abdomen. Which one of the following organisms is the most likely cause of her traveller's diarrhoea?

☐ A   *Enterococcus faecalis*
☐ B   Enterotoxigenic *Escherichia coli*
☐ C   *Salmonella typhi*
☐ D   *Salmonella paratyphi*
☐ E   *Clostridium difficile*

28. Which of the following is true of *Cryptosporidium parvum* infection?

☐ A   It is spread by droplet infection
☐ B   It can be detected by staining stool for acid-fast bacilli
☐ C   Chlorination of drinking water supplies has markedly reduced infection rates
☐ D   It produces severe disease in most infected individuals
☐ E   It is treated with a prolonged course of metronidazole

29. Which one of the following pairings of pathogen and appropriate therapeutic agents is correct?

☐ A   *Fasciola hepatica* – praziquantel
☐ B   *Aspergillus fumigatus* – ketoconazole
☐ C   *Toxoplasma gondii* – primaquine
☐ D   *Strongyloides stercoralis* – ivermectin
☐ E   *Onchocerca volvulus* – quinacrine

30. **By which one of these processes may DNA be transferred naturally among bacteria?**

☐ A Recombination
☐ B Translocation
☐ C Transcription
☐ D Mutation
☐ E Conjugation

31. **Which one of the following is true of recombinant hepatitis B vaccine?**

☐ A At best it offers around 70% protection against disease
☐ B It is a whole virus vaccine
☐ C It offers some cross-protection against hepatitis A
☐ D It has a lower response rate in patients with diabetes mellitus
☐ E It may cause arthritis in patients who already have anti-HBs antibodies

32. **To which one of the following is HIV highly resistant?**

☐ A Autoclave
☐ B Chlorhexidine
☐ C Hot air oven
☐ D Hypochlorites
☐ E Gluteraldehyde

33. **Which one of the following pairings of infection and transmission route is correct?**

☐ A Ebola virus – infected rhesus monkeys
☐ B *Leishmania tropica* – blackfly
☐ C *Trypanosoma cruzi* – exposure to contaminated freshwater lakes
☐ D Katayama fever – *Aedes* species of mosquito
☐ E *Herpesvirus simiae* (B virus) – blood transfusions

34. Which one of the following antiviral agents is correctly matched with the site of inhibition of viral replication?

☐ A Zidovudine – translation of viral proteins
☐ B Ganciclovir – uncoating of RNA in the cell
☐ C Amantadine – viral DNA polymerase
☐ D Interferon – viral protein synthesis
☐ E Stavudine – HIV protease

35. Which one of the following may depend on human rather than vertebrate animal hosts in their primary transmission cycle?

☐ A Japanese encephalitis
☐ B Tick-borne encephalitis
☐ C Dengue fever
☐ D St Louis encephalitis
☐ E Hantavirus pulmonary syndrome

36. A 46-year-old sheep-farmer is admitted to hospital with a six-week history of fevers and progressive breathlessness. On examination, he has two splinter haemorrhages on his left hand, hepatosplenomegaly, and a grade 3/6 pansystolic murmur, which is thought to be new. An echocardiogram confirms a large mitral valve vegetation with moderate mitral regurgitation. He is commenced on intravenous benzylpenicillin and gentamicin after three sets of blood cultures have been sent. Despite a week of antimicrobial therapy, his fevers continue and a total of six sets of blood cultures have failed to yield an organism. Which one of the following organisms is likely to be the cause of his endocarditis?

☐ A Methicillin-resistant *Staphylococcus aureus*
☐ B *Candida albicans*
☐ C *Coxiella burnetii*
☐ D *Streptococcus viridans*
☐ E *Enterococcus faecalis*

37. A 34-year-old soldier is airlifted from Iraq after sustaining a landmine injury. He is admitted to an Intensive Care Unit with full-thickness burns to his torso and lower limbs. He undergoes extensive surgical debridement and reconstruction, and appears to be recovering well. On day 6 after admission, however, he begins to spike fevers and his ventilatory requirements increase dramatically. Blood cultures become positive for a Gram-negative coccobacillus, which is resistant to meropenem, ceftazidime and Tazocin®. Over the next two days, the same organism is cultured from what are usually sterile sites in several other patients. Which one of the following organisms is the likely cause?

- [ ] A Pseudomonas aeruginosa
- [ ] B Acinetobacter baumanii
- [ ] C Neisseria meningitidis
- [ ] D Methicillin-resistant Staphylococcus aureus
- [ ] E Aeromonas hydrophila

38. A 72-year-old woman is admitted to hospital from a nursing home with worsening cellulitis of her right leg, which has originated from a venous ulcer. She has had multiple similar episodes in the past and a swab of the ulcer six months previously had grown methicillin-resistant Staphylococcus aureus (MRSA). She is commenced on intravenous vancomycin, the dose being adjusted according to levels over the next two days. Despite this therapy, she becomes more unwell and an MRSA is cultured from her blood. To which one of the following antimicrobials may she respond?

- [ ] A Linezolid
- [ ] B Tazocin®
- [ ] C Teicoplanin
- [ ] D Ceftazidime
- [ ] E Rifampicin

39. Eight years ago a 25-year-old intravenous drug user was admitted to hospital with a maculopapular rash, neck-stiffness, headache and a sore throat. A CT scan of his head and lumbar puncture were performed, which were both unremarkable apart from a mild CSF lymphocytosis (8 cells/mm^3). His symptoms resolved over the next few days and he was discharged with a provisional diagnosis of viral meningitis. He has now been readmitted to hospital with a four-week history of headaches and vomiting. A CT scan of his head is normal and a lumbar puncture is performed, which reveals an opening pressure of 30 cmH$_2$O and positive India ink staining consistent with *Cryptococcus neoformans*. An HIV test is performed which is positive. Which one of the following best describes the probable Centers for Disease Control (CDC) stages of HIV infection which he presented with during his two admissions to hospital?

- [ ] A   Stage 2 and stage 3
- [ ] B   Stage 1 and stage 2
- [ ] C   Stage 2 and stage 4
- [ ] D   Stage 1 and stage 4
- [ ] E   Stage 1 and stage 3

40. A 29-year-old British nurse has returned from Ethiopia after a six-month secondment with Médicins Sans Frontières. She was taking mefloquine as malaria prophylaxis but stopped due to side effects. She presents with a three-day history of fevers. A blood film shows the presence of *Plasmodium vivax* infection. Which one of the following combinations would be the most appropriate treatment?

- [ ] A   Quinine and primaquine
- [ ] B   Quinine and Fansidar®
- [ ] C   Quinine and Doxycycline
- [ ] D   Chloroquine and primaquine
- [ ] E   Chloroquine and Fansidar®

MICROBIOLOGY

Answers

1.   **A: It has a polysaccharide capsule**

Neisseria meningitidis is a Gram-negative diplococcus with a polysaccharide capsule. It may be detected in CSF using a latex agglutination test. It is part of the normal oropharyngeal flora and is found in 20–40% of healthy young adults. During epidemics of meningococcal disease in institutionalised populations, colonisation rates may approach 90%. It dies quickly at room temperature outside the human host. The meningococcal vaccine contains capsular polysaccharides of A, C, Y and W-135 strains, but no vaccine is currently available for group B strains (which are responsible for 70% of cases of meningococcal septicaemia in the UK). The Waterhouse–Friderichsen syndrome is adrenal haemorrhage secondary to meningococcal septicaemia.

2.   **E: It causes meningitis**

Listeria monocytogenes is a catalase-positive, Gram-positive diplococcus. It is susceptible to ampicillin. Infection usually follows the ingestion of contaminated food, especially unpasteurised dairy products. Problems usually only occur in pregnant women and in immunocompromised patients. In the pregnant mother the infection is self-limiting but it can affect the child, causing stillbirth, septic abortion, premature delivery, pneumonia and meningoencephalitis. Group B *Streptococcus* is the other main causative agent of neonatal bacteraemia. It is also a Gram-positive diplococcus and may be confused with *Listeria monocytogenes* on Gram-staining. They can be easily distinguished on Gram-stain, however, as group B *Streptococcus* is catalase-negative.

3. **C: Organisms causing systemic infection are usually encapsulated**

    Haemophilus influenzae is a small, Gram-negative, non-motile rod. It may cause meningitis, pneumonia, otitis media, sinusitis and, rarely, epiglottitis. Organisms which cause systemic infection are nearly always encapsulated, most commonly with type b polysaccharide. A conjugated vaccine has been developed against this, coupled with either diphtheria or tetanus toxoid. This combination vaccine is now used in infants with the initial series of vaccinations at two, four and six months of age. Amoxicillin is used in the treatment and rifampicin in the prophylaxis of *H. influenzae* infections.

4. **B: *Neisseria meningitidis***

    Penicillin is active against most aerobic Gram-positive organisms. It is not effective against most Gram-negative rods, such as *H. influenzae*, *E. coli*, and *P. aeruginosa*, though ampicillin and amoxicillin have some activity. Penicillin is also inactive against bacterial cells which are not growing.

5. **C: Flavivirus – yellow fever**

    Rotaviruses cause infantile diarrhoea and upper respiratory tract infections. Lassa fever is due to an arenavirus. Both Lassa fever and Ebola virus disease are due to arenaviruses with a high person-to-person transmission rate and a relatively high case fertility rate. Flaviviruses cause yellow and dengue fevers. When first discovered, HIV-1 was classified as 'HTLV-3'.

6. **D: The presence of anti-HBs in the serum indicates immunity**

    Appearance of anti-HBs in the serum usually signifies a successful recovery from infection. Clinical recovery and clearance of the virus is associated with the disappearance of HBeAg and then HBsAg, with subsequent detection of their respective antibodies during recovery. The 'e' antigen is a marker of infectivity. The risk of transmission with a needlestick injury from a HbsAg-positive source is approximately 30%. Hepatitis B virus is present in the saliva and semen of infected persons.

7. **A: Seroconversion following HIV infection generally occurs 3–12 weeks after exposure**

Seroconversion following HIV infection generally occurs 3–12 weeks after infection. There is an association between the acquisition of HIV and a number of sexually transmitted diseases (STDs), especially ulcerated STDs (eg syphilis, chancroid). The envelope of HIV contains two linked glycoproteins, gp120 and gp41, cleaved from a common precursor, gp160. The p24 and p17 glycoproteins are two of the four proteins that make up the nucleocapsid of HIV (the others are p9 and p7) and are cleaved from p53, encoded by the *gag* gene.

Primary HIV infection may be symptomatic in as many as 50–90% of cases after initial exposure to HIV. Symptoms usually occur two to four weeks after infection, coinciding with the acute widespread dissemination of the virus. Symptoms persist for four weeks and start to resolve with the decline in HIV viral load and the development of cytotoxic T lymphocytes and HIV-specific antibodies.

Laboratory evaluation within the first two weeks of acute HIV infection is characterised by lymphopenia, with reduction of both the CD4 and CD8 cell subsets. The CD4 cell count during this period may decrease to < 200 cells/mm^3. Four or more weeks after infection, there is a dramatic increase in CD8 and, to lesser extent, CD4 cells, leading to a sustained inversion of the CD4:CD8 ratio. Disease progression is therefore associated with a fall in the CD4:CD8 ratio, but a rise in β_2-microglobulin (a marker of immune activation).

8. **C: It is sensitive to erythromycin**

Legionella pneumophila is a slender Gram-negative rod (which stains poorly) and is found in up to 75% of water cooling systems. There is no case-to-case transmission. Diagnosis is made by detecting a significant rise in antibody titre by use of indirect immunofluorescence. A rise in cold agglutinins and haemolytic anaemia may be found in atypical pneumonia caused by mycoplasma.

9. D: *Salmonella* species

Patients with sickle cell disease are at a greatly increased risk of infection from encapsulated organisms, including *Pneumococcus, Haemophilus influenzae,* type B meningococcus and *Salmonella enteritidis.* Vaccination and antibiotic prophylaxis should be employed. In addition to pneumonia, bacteraemia and meningitis, osteomyelitis (mainly due to *Salmonella* species) is a problem in these patients. Osteomyelitis usually affects the long bones and *Staphylococcus aureus,* the usual causative agent in non-sickle cell patients, accounts for fewer than 25% of cases.

10. E: Congenital cataracts may be seen in affected neonates

The congenital rubella syndrome consists of:

1. Cardiac defects – patent ductus arteriosus, coarctation of the aorta, pulmonary stenosis
2. Ophthalmic defects – retinopathy, congenital cataracts, glaucoma, choroidoretinitis
3. Endocrine defects – diabetes mellitus, growth retardation, thyroid disease
4. Renal defects – renal artery stenosis, polycystic kidney disease
5. CNS defects – encephalopathy, microencephalopathy, sensorineural deafness
6. Reticuloendothelial defects – bony lesions on X-ray, hepatosplenomegaly, thrombocytopenia.

The risk to the fetus is about 90% if the mother has rubella during the first trimester. Sensorineural deafness tends to occur, however, if the fetus is affected between 11–16 weeks, after which the risk is very low. Babies with the congenital rubella syndrome excrete virus for long periods – often for more than three months. During this time they are highly infectious. The diagnosis can be made on raised specific IgM titres from cord blood or by direct culture from throat or eye swabs, urine or stool.

11. D: Infantile eczema

Specific contraindications to routine vaccination include: febrile illness or intercurrent infection; hypersensitivity to egg protein (contraindication to influenza vaccine); previous anaphylactic reaction to egg (contraindication to measles/mumps/rubella, influenza and yellow fever vaccines); infantile eczema. No live vaccine should be given in immunodeficiency or with immunosuppressive therapy (including high-dose steroids), in malignancy, or in pregnancy.

12. A: The appearance of calcification on the skull X-ray

Toxoplasma gondii infection is generally asymptomatic in the mother when it is contracted during pregnancy. Toxoplasmosis has widespread effects on the developing brain, causing hydrocephalus, microcephaly, cerebral calcification, and a choroidoretinitis. There is usually a resultant mental handicap. If the pregnant woman was infected before conception there is no risk of transmission to the fetus. For maternal toxoplasmosis acquired during pregnancy, the risk of congenital toxoplasmosis is 14% during the first trimester, 29% during the second trimester, and 59% during the third trimester (ie the risk doubles with each trimester).

13. C: It does not grow well anaerobically

Escherichia coli is an aerobic, lactose-fermenting, non-spore-forming Gram-negative rod. Vancomycin is mainly active against Gram-positive organisms; gentamicin should be used in severe *E. coli* sepsis.

14. E: There is an equal incidence in men and women

Creutzfeldt–Jakob disease (CJD) is caused by a transmissible prion protein. Cases of infection following corneal transplant or the accidental introduction of infected reticuloendothelial or brain tissue have been reported. The familial form is responsible for only 15% of cases. Men and women are affected equally. It is mainly a disease of age, but variant CJD affects younger patients. Brain pathology shows a spongiform encephalopathy with amyloid deposition and vacuolation, but demyelination does not occur.

15. C: Brucellosis

Infections acquired from animal sources:

Organism	Disease or infection	Source
Borrelia burgdorferi	Lyme disease	Birds, deer, mammals
Listeria monocytogenes	Listeriosis	Sheep, cattle
Brucella spp.	Brucellosis	Cattle, sheep, swine, dogs
Toxoplasma gondii	Toxoplasmosis	Cats
Leptospira spp.	Leptospirosis	Dogs, rats, cattle
Yersinia pestis	Plague	Rats
Francisella tularensis	Tularaemia	Deer, rabbits

Cholera is caused by a bacterial exotoxin. Trichomoniasis is a sexually transmitted protozoal infection.

16. E: *Corynebacterium diphtheriae*

Extracellular exotoxins are produced by most Gram-positive bacteria. In addition, they are also produced by some Gram-negative organisms (*Vibrio cholerae*, *Shigella* spp.). *Escherichia coli* O157 produces the verotoxin which causes haemolytic-uraemic syndrome. The exotoxin produced in diphtheria causes cardiotoxicity and neurotoxicity.

17. B: *Mycobacterium tuberculosis*

Asymptomatic carriage of *Mycobacterium tuberculosis* is rare, but small numbers of organisms may lie dormant in unhealed lesions. *S. pyogenes* may be present in the upper respiratory tract in 5–10% of healthy people.

18. A: Cholecystitis

Cholecystitis is caused by superinfection with normal gut flora. Toxic shock syndrome is mediated by a toxin produced by some strains of *Staphylococcus aureus*. Toxic epidermal necrolysis is due to splitting of desmosomes by exfoliative toxins of the group II serotypes 55 and 71. Some strains of *S. aureus* produce an enterotoxin which can cause food poisoning.

19. C: Person-to-person transmission is the major route of spread

Beta-lactam-resistant *Staphylococcus aureus* is an important cause of community-acquired and nosocomial infections. Beta-lactam-resistant strains are uniformly resistant to penicillin, ampicillin, amoxicillin and methicillin. It is thought that β-lactam-resistant isolates are at least as virulent as susceptible strains, if not more so. In large hospital outbreaks, patient-to-patient spread is mostly via hospital staff who carry the organism on their hands. Most strains are coagulase-positive and catalase-negative.

20. D: BCG

It is not safe to give live vaccines to potentially immunocompromised patients. Measles vaccine may be less effective in HIV-positive patients, and administration of normal human immunoglobulin following contact with measles should be considered. There have been reports of generalised BCG infection in HIV-infected patients.

21. D: It has a prevalence of up to 90% in haemophiliacs

Hepatitis C virus (HCV) is a single-stranded RNA virus. It is transmitted parenterally by intravenous drug abuse (40%), by sexual contact (10%) or via transfusion of infected blood products (10%). The route of infection is unidentified in about 40% of cases. Anti-HCV antibody is detected in the serum by immunoblot assays, which are highly sensitive and specific. Around 50% of patients with acute hepatitis C will develop chronic hepatitis, and 20% of these will develop cirrhosis, with its risk of progression to hepatocellular carcinoma. Interferon-α-2b, either alone or in combination with riboflavin, has been shown to normalise or near-normalise ALT levels in 50% of patients, with an associated reduction or elimination of HCV RNA from the serum. However, 50% of responders relapse within six months of dicontinuing treatment.

22. E: The standard vaccine is rarely effective in children under the age of six years

Streptococcus pneumoniae has at least 80 serotypes. The current vaccine contains the 23 serotypes which most commonly cause disease. *S. pneumoniae* may cause acute endocarditis and pericarditis, but it is *Streptococcus viridans* which is most commonly associated with subacute bacterial endocarditis. *S. pneumoniae* may develop some resistance to penicillin, but this is due to a change in the penicillin-binding proteins in the cell wall rather than to β-lactamase production. Individuals with sickle cell disease have a 600-fold increase in the risk of severe pneumococcal sepsis. The full potential for mounting an immunological response to polysaccharide agents is not reached until around the age of six years, but a new conjugate vaccine is now available for infants.

23. D: It causes erythema infectiosum

Parvovirus B19 is a DNA virus. It is usually acquired in childhood, between the ages of four and ten years, and serological evidence of infection may be found in 40–60% of the adult population. It is the cause of erythema infectiosum (fifth disease) in children. Parvovirus B19 causes persistent anaemia in immunocompromised individuals as a result of bone marrow suppression, and aplastic crises in patients with chronic haemolytic anaemia.

24. **A: The causative organism is found in the mucus which lines the gastric epithelium**

Helicobacter pylori is a Gram-negative bacterium which is found in 90% of patients with duodenal ulcers and in 70% of patients with gastric ulceration. The urease breath test, using urea labelled with ^{14}C is a useful aid to diagnosis. Serum antibodies may remain detectable more than six months after successful eradication.

25. **B: Phenoxymethylpenicillin**

Phenoxymethylpenicillin (penicillin V) is destroyed by β-lactamase. Other agents which would be effective in treating this infection include cefuroxime and septrin, which are both resistant to the action of β-lactamase.

26. **E: It may cause infective endocarditis**

The enterococci are forms of streptococci which are part of the normal gut flora. They may also be found on the skin, and in the oropharyx and genitourinary tract. They are an important cause of nosocomial infection in patients with indwelling catheters, and of endocarditis in patients with abnormal or prosthetic heart valves. They are frequently isolated, with other organisms, from intra-abdominal abscesses and wound infections. They are much less sensitive to penicillin than other streptococci. They do not cause haemolysis.

27. **B: Enterotoxigenic *Escherichia coli***

One-third to a half of all cases of traveller's diarrhoea is caused by enterotoxigenic *E. coli*. Enteroinvasive *E. coli* and *Shigella* each account for less than 10%, while amoebiasis accounts for less than 5%. The frequency of *Giardia* infection varies widely with the area visited. *Salmonella typhi* and *Salmonella paratyphi* are causes of enteric fever, a septic febrile illness in which diarrhoea is a late feature. *Clostridium difficile* causes pseudomembranous colitis.

28. B: It can be detected by staining stool for acid-fast bacilli (AFB)

Crytosporidium parvum is spread via contact with infected water supplies or affected individuals or animals. It is diagnosed by finding cysts in stool or biopsy material. A modified AFB smear will demonstrate the organism and is a useful diagnostic aid. The organism is highly resistant to chlorination. It causes a mild to severe, self-limiting illness in healthy people, but may be life-threatening in the immunocompromised. There is no specific effective therapy. HIV-infected individuals are advised to boil their drinking water.

29. D: *Strongyloides stercoralis* – ivermectin

Fasciola hepatica, the sheep liver fluke, and *Onchocerca volvulus*, the cause of river blindness, are both treated with ivermectin. *Aspergillus* is best treated with amphotericin, but itraconazole has some activity. Toxoplasmosis is treated with a combination of pyrimethamine and sulfadoxine or sulfadiazine. *Strongyloides stercoralis* infection is acquired from larvae which reside in the wall of the small intestine following infection; a cycle of autoinfection may occur.

30. E: Conjugation

True recombination only occurs in diploid cells during meiosis. Translocation and transcription are steps in protein synthesis and do not relate to direct transfer of DNA between bacteria. Mutation is the change in nucleotide sequence in DNA. Conjugation is the mating and direct transfer of DNA (a plasmid or resistance factor) between bacterial cells in contact. An example is the development of gentamicin resistance. Transduction refers to the transfer of DNA via viruses which infect bacteria (bacteriophages), for example the development of penicillin resistance by *Staphylococcus aureus*.

31. D: It has a lower response rate in patients with diabetes mellitus

The recombinant hepatitis B vaccine (HBvaxPRO® or Engerix B®) is highly effective (around 90%) in protecting against hepatitis B infection, but offers no cross-protection against other hepatitis viruses. It is a subunit vaccine, containing the HBs antigen but not the viral core. The response rate is lower in patients with diabetes (70–80%), HIV infection (50–70%), renal failure (60–70%) or chronic liver disease (60–70%). There is no increased incidence in side effects when administered to a patient who already has HbsAg antibodies. The other factors associated with a suboptimal response to hepatitis B vaccine are obesity, viral 'escape' mutants, and older age.

32. B: Chlorhexidine

Chlorhexidine is active against most bacteria apart from *Mycobacterium tuberculosis*, but has limited activity against viruses and bacterial spores. Gluteraldehyde is effective against many viruses, including HIV and hepatitis B, and against bacterial spores, but gluteraldehyde should only be used when other alternatives are not available. Hypochlorite is effective against hepatitis B virus, HIV, other viruses, and some bacteria.

33. A: Ebola virus – infected rhesus monkeys

African rhesus monkeys have recently been reported to have Ebola virus infection. The rhesus monkey is also thought to be the source of herpesvirus simiae (B virus). *Leishmania tropica* is carried by the sandfly; river blindness (onchocerciasis) is spread by blackfly. *Trypanosoma cruzi* causes Chagas' disease and is carried by the reduviid insect (the 'kissing bug'). Katayama fever is acute schistosomiasis and is acquired by contact with freshwater harbouring the parasite.

34. D: Interferon – viral protein synthesis

Zidovudine and stavudine are nucleoside reverse transcriptase inhibitors (NRTIs). Ganciclovir inhibits viral DNA polymerase following phosphorylation by CMV-induced kinases. Amantadine inhibits uncoating of the virus in the cell. Interferon works by inhibiting:

- viral penetration or uncoating
- synthesis of messenger RNA
- translation of viral proteins
- viral assembly and release.

35. C: Dengue fever

Dengue fever is mainly maintained in a human–mosquito–human cycle, although monkeys may be involved. Tick-borne encephalitis is transmitted between ticks and rodents, and St Louis encephalitis involves mosquitoes, and birds and pigs. Hantaviruses are single-stranded enveloped viruses which are related to members of the Bunyaviridae family. Hantavirus vectors are mostly rodents: fieldmice and dormice, voles and rats. Infected rodents shed infectious virions from aerosolised urine or faeces, and the main route of transmission is via inhalation of these shed virions.

36. C: *Coxiella burnetii*

Coxiella burnetii is an atypical bacterium that only replicates intracellularly. It is the only member of the genus *Coxiella* and is a cause of culture-negative endocarditis and Q fever. It is transmitted to humans from sheep and cattle, mainly by inhalation of contaminated dust or via infected placenta at parturition. Diagnosis is by serological testing and treatment of the endocarditis requires long-term doxycycline and ciprofloxacin or rifamipicin. Other causes of culture-negative endocarditis include *Chlamydia psittaci* infection, recent antibiotic therapy, and infection with fastidious organisms (eg HACEK group organisms).

37. B: *Acinetobacter baumanii*

Acinetobacter baumanii is an opportunistic pathogen seen in patients with ventilator-associated pneumonia and catheter-related septicaemia in the Intensive Care Unit setting. It is widely distributed in nature and may be an insignificant finding in wounds and sputum. In contrast, it is usually pathogenic when recovered from sterile sites. It is usually sensitive to carbapenems (imipenem, meropenem), although some multi-drug-resistant strains have recently caused outbreaks in the UK.

38. A: Linezolid

Linezolid is a new oxazolidinone antibiotic, which is available in both intravenous and oral forms. It is active against both methicillin-resistant *S. aureus* and vancomycin-resistant *Enterococcus*. Serious side effects include thrombocytopenia and anaemia (dose-dependent and reversible) and, rarely, lactic acidosis.

39. D: Stage 1 and stage 4

Stage 1 – primary infection: around 25–65% have an illness at seroconversion. This is usually a mild mononucleosis-like illness two weeks to three months after exposure, with a fever, maculopapular rash, sore throat, lymphadenopathy, night sweats and diarrhoea. It may include genital and mouth ulcers, as well as neurological features such as encephalopathy, meningitis and myelopathy.

Stage 2 – asymptomatic infection: of variable duration (one to ten years), the CD4 count is usually over 350 cells/mm^3 and the HIV RNA level (viral load) is low.

Stage 3 – syptomatic disease: viral replication increases and the CD4 count declines. There is malaise, weight loss, fever, night sweats and opportunistic infections occur.

Stage 4 – AIDS: usually correlated with a CD4 count of less than 200 cells/mm^3.

Cryptococcal meningitis usually occurs when CD4 counts are less than 100 cells/mm^3.

40. D: Chloroquine and primaquine

Plasmodium vivax, unlike *P. falciparum,* is still chloroquine-sensitive in most parts of the world. Some resistance has been reported from South America and Oceania. *P. vivax* and *P. ovale* both have a liver hypnozoite stage which can result in relapses years later. Most of the drugs used in malaria prophylaxis and treatment are blood schizonticides, with the exception of primaquine, which is active against the liver stage. In those with *P. vivax* or *P. ovale* infection, G6PD deficiency should be excluded (as primaquine can cause haemolysis in this condition) and a 14-day course of primaquine should be given after treatment of the acute disease.

Chapter 4

IMMUNOLOGY

Questions

1. A 54-year-old woman has end-stage renal failure secondary to adult polycystic kidney disease. She has undergone thrice-weekly haemodialysis for several years, and has been on the transplant waiting list for 18 months. A potential donor organ becomes available following the death of a 23-year-old woman in a road traffic accident. Tissue typing is still pending. Which one of the following is true of cadaveric renal transplantation?

☐ A Both CD4 and CD8 cells mediate acute rejection following transplantation

☐ B DRw6-negative grafts have a better outcome than DRw6-positive grafts

☐ C Multiple blood transfusions prior to grafting increases the likelihood of graft rejection

☐ D Matching for MHC class I antigens is more important than matching for class II antigens in determining graft survival

☐ E The main effect of ciclosporin A is on CD8 cell-dependent proliferative responses

2. Which one of the following is true regarding the major histocompatibility complex?

☐ A It is located on the short arm of chromosome 4

☐ B Class II antigens are coded for by A, B and C genes

☐ C Class II antigens are more crucial to graft survival than ABO blood group compatibility

☐ D Matching at the A and C loci has the greatest influence on graft survival

☐ E Non-identical siblings have a 2:4 chance of sharing two antigens

3. A mother takes her young daughter to visit her general practitioner because the little girl has a rash on her neck which is inflamed and itchy. On taking a careful history, it is discovered that the child received a necklace as a gift around one month ago. Which one of the following is true of this type of hypersensitivity reaction?

- [ ] A   It is dependent on complement
- [ ] B   It is dependent on B lymphocytes
- [ ] C   It is independent of antibody
- [ ] D   It is more common in HIV-infected patients
- [ ] E   It is responsible for autoimmune haemolytic anaemia

4. Which one of the following is an example of a type V hypersensitivity reaction?

- [ ] A   Hyperacute rejection of a transplanted kidney
- [ ] B   Haemolysis following a blood transfusion
- [ ] C   Haemolytic anaemia due to *Mycoplasma pneumoniae*
- [ ] D   Hyperthyroidism in Graves' disease
- [ ] E   Idiopathic thrombocytopenia

5. Which one of the following is a major immunological abnormality in advanced HIV infection?

- [ ] A   Marked lymphopenia, especially of cells bearing the CD8 cell marker
- [ ] B   Polyclonal B-cell activation
- [ ] C   Increased natural killer cell activity
- [ ] D   A fall in the CD8:CD4 ratio in the peripheral blood
- [ ] E   A hyperacute cutaneous hypersensitivity response

6. **Which one of the following occurs in an HIV-infected individual?**

☐ A   Soluble CD4 molecules bind to HIV and block its infectivity
☐ B   The diagnosis of HIV is usually confirmed by positive isolation and culture
☐ C   The first antibodies to appear after infection are directed against core proteins
☐ D   Ciclosporin A inhibits reverse transcriptase
☐ E   Skin tests to common antigens are usually exaggerated

7. **A 38-year-old woman is referred to the Rheumatology Outpatients Department. She has a two-month history of stiffness in her fingers, toes and wrists, lasting around two hours in the mornings. A diagnosis of rheumatoid arthritis is suspected, and a serum sample is positive for rheumatoid factor. Which one of the following is true of rheumatoid factor?**

☐ A   It is found in 50% of patients with SLE
☐ B   It must be present for the diagnosis of rheumatoid arthritis
☐ C   It is directed against the Fc fragment of the patient's own IgM
☐ D   It is usually IgM
☐ E   It is only found in patients with connective tissue disease

8. **Which one of the following diseases is most likely to result in low complement levels?**

☐ A   Rheumatoid arthritis
☐ B   Ankylosing spondylitis
☐ C   Systemic lupus erythematosus (SLE)
☐ D   Systemic sclerosis
☐ E   Sjögren's syndrome

Answers on pages 82–84   71

9. **Which one of the following statements is true?**

☐ A B lymphocytes are characterised by rosette formation with sheep red cells
☐ B T cells make up 70% of circulating lymphocytes
☐ C IgE makes up around 10% of the total immunoglobulins in the serum
☐ D Rheumatoid factor is an acute phase protein
☐ E IgG and IgE are the only antibodies small enough to cross the placenta

10. **Hypogammaglobulinaemia can be a feature in which one of the following diseases?**

☐ A Tuberculosis
☐ B Sarcoidosis
☐ C Kala-azar
☐ D Malaria
☐ E Subacute endocarditis

11. **A 41-year-old female patient presents with a history of difficulty swallowing. She also tells the doctor that she suffers from painful fingers when it is cold, and that she has little lumps in the palms of her hands and at the back of her ankles. An underlying connective tissue disease is suspected. The serum antinuclear antibody (ANA) is markedly raised. In which one of the following conditions is ANA usually absent?**

☐ A Sjögren's syndrome
☐ B Polyarteritis nodosa
☐ C Scleroderma
☐ D Infective endocarditis
☐ E Rheumatoid arthritis

12. **Soluble circulating immune complexes may be found in which one of the following conditions?**

☐ A Dermatitis herpetiformis
☐ B Rhesus haemolytic disease
☐ C Post-streptococcal glomerulonephritis
☐ D Tuberculosis
☐ E Myasthenia gravis

13. **In which one of the following conditions is the delayed hypersensitivity reaction preserved?**

☐ A Wiscott–Aldrich syndrome
☐ B Malnutrition
☐ C Sarcoidosis
☐ D Hodgkin's disease
☐ E Scleroderma

14. **Which of the following is true of tumour necrosis factor (TNF)?**

☐ A It reduces capillary permeability
☐ B It is the predominant cause of shock in Gram-negative septicaemia
☐ C It causes toxic shock syndrome
☐ D It has no role in the host response to viruses
☐ E It causes natural killer (NK) cells to release interferon-α

15. **You work in a centre which receives referrals from the local public health consultant for the testing and immunisation of patients with recent tuberculosis contacts or those with abnormal Mantoux tests. Which one of the following people should not receive BCG?**

☐ A An adult immigrant from Bangladesh
☐ B A Mantoux-negative healthcare worker
☐ C A Mantoux-positive schoolchild
☐ D A seven-year-old immigrant child from Bangladesh
☐ E A neonate whose grandmother has active TB

Answers on pages 84–86

16. Which one of the following statements about IgA is true?

☐ A It has a key role in mucosal immunity
☐ B It has four distinct subgroups
☐ C It activates complement via the classical pathway
☐ D It is manufactured in the lymph nodes
☐ E It crosses the placenta

17. A 24-year-old man with a long-term history of asthma is referred by his general practitioner to the Respiratory Outpatients Clinic. Despite taking maximal doses of inhaled steroids and a long-acting β_2-agonist, his asthma is still poorly controlled. You consider starting him on Montelukast (leukotriene receptor antagonist). Which one of the following is true of leukotrienes?

☐ A They are produced and released mainly by lymphocytes
☐ B Their breakdown results in the formation of arachidonic acid
☐ C They decrease vascular permeability
☐ D They include the slow-reacting substance of anaphylaxis (SRS-A)
☐ E They cause bronchodilatation

18. Which one of the following is true of the acute phase response?

☐ A It causes a reduction in plasma viscosity
☐ B It is particularly marked in viral infections
☐ C It may be assessed by measurement of C peptide
☐ D It is stimulated by cytokines
☐ E It is characterised by the breakdown of proteins in the liver

19. Which one of the following is associated with the presence of cytoplasmic-staining antineutrophil cytoplasmic antibodies (c-ANCA)?

☐ A Scleroderma
☐ B Microscopic polyarteritis
☐ C SLE
☐ D Rheumatoid arthritis
☐ E Wegener's granulomatosis

20. **In which one of the following conditions could treatment with intravenous immunoglobulin result in an adverse outcome?**

- [ ] A The acquired immunodeficiency syndrome in a child
- [ ] B Chronic lymphocytic leukaemia
- [ ] C Isolated IgA deficiency
- [ ] D X-linked hypogammaglobulinaemia
- [ ] E Guillain–Barré syndrome

21. **Which one of the following is true of immunoglobulin M?**

- [ ] A It is predominantly extravascular
- [ ] B It has eight antigen-binding sites
- [ ] C Its concentration is increased in the serum of patients with untreated coeliac disease
- [ ] D It is responsible for the determination of blood group
- [ ] E It has a half-life of ten days

22. **Which one of the following conditions is most characteristically associated with Bruton's congenital agammaglobulinaemia?**

- [ ] A Neonatal sepsis
- [ ] B Tonsillar hypertrophy
- [ ] C Meningoencephalitis due to echovirus infection
- [ ] D Mucocutaenous candidiasis
- [ ] E Aspergillosis

23. **Which one of the following is most true of interferons?**

- [ ] A They are virus proteins that inhibit activation of T cells
- [ ] B They act within infected cells to inhibit virus replication
- [ ] C They are the principal mediators in the host response to Gram-negative bacteria
- [ ] D Interferon-α leads to the suppression of helper T-2 (T_H2) cells
- [ ] E Interferon-β leads to enhanced MHC class II expression

24. **Which one of the following features is characteristic of the primary antiphospholipid syndrome?**

- [ ] A   The ratio of female to male cases is 9:1
- [ ] B   It generally presents earlier than systemic lupus erythematosus
- [ ] C   Recurrent fetal loss is the commonest presentation
- [ ] D   Antibodies to double-stranded DNA (dsDNA) are present in more than 60% of patients
- [ ] E   The prolonged clotting time does not correct with normal plasma

25. **Which one of the following organisms uses antigenic variation as a major means of evading host defences?**

- [ ] A   *Streptococcus pneumoniae*
- [ ] B   *Mycobacterium tuberculosis*
- [ ] C   Hepatitis C virus
- [ ] D   *Haemophilus influenzae*
- [ ] E   *Trypanosoma brucei*

26. **Which one of the following statements about interferon-γ (IFN-γ) is true?**

- [ ] A   It is useful in the treatment of chronic hepatitis B infection
- [ ] B   It is useful in treating chronic hepatitis C infection
- [ ] C   It is useful in the treatment of chronic granulomatous disease
- [ ] D   It is useful in the management of malignant melanoma
- [ ] E   It is therapeutically useful in hairy cell leukaemia

27. **Which one of the following reactions is characteristic of a type-2 helper T cell (T$_H$2) response?**

- [ ] A   IL-2 secretion
- [ ] B   Production of IgE
- [ ] C   Development of a granuloma
- [ ] D   A cell-mediated immune response
- [ ] E   Interferon-γ production

28. **Which one of the following is true of antimitochondrial antibodies?**

☐ A They are found in nearly all patients with primary biliary cirrhosis

☐ B They are found in 20% of patients with SLE

☐ C They are responsible for the bile duct damage seen in primary biliary cirrhosis

☐ D They are associated with the presence of the HLA-A1_1-B8_1-DR3 haplotype

☐ E They are frequently accompanied by a rise in IgM antibodies in patients with chronic active hepatitis

29. **Which one of the following statements about MHC class II molecules is true?**

☐ A They are expressed on almost all nucleated cells

☐ B There is minimal variability between siblings

☐ C They are coded for by the genes HLA-A, -B and -C

☐ D They act as receptors for the presentation of antigen to helper T cells

☐ E They are the main reason for graft rejection between siblings

30. **Which one of the following cells is involved in the initial presentation of antigen to T cells?**

☐ A Monocytes

☐ B Neutrophils

☐ C Follicular dendritic cells

☐ D CD8 cells

☐ E Red cells

Answers on pages 89–92

31. A patient is seen in the Dermatology Clinic with a three-month history of an itchy rash affecting the face and trunk. The diagnosis is not immediately apparent on examination, so a skin biopsy is taken. Which one of the following skin conditions is matched with the correct finding on direct immunofluorescent examination of a skin biopsy?

☐ A Pemphigoid – autoantibodies to epidermal intracellular cement
☐ B Pemphigus – granular IgA deposits in the dermal papillae
☐ C Dermatitis herpetiformis – autoantibodies to epidermal intercellular cement
☐ D SLE – deposits of immunoglobulin and complement along the basement membrane zone
☐ E SLE – deposits of immunoglobulins at the dermal-epidermal junction of unaffected skin in the lupus band test

32. A 54-year-old woman with chronic obstructive pulmonary disease is admitted to hospital with a two-day history of worsening dyspnoea and fever and a cough productive of green sputum. A chest X-ray reveals right lower lobe consolidation. She has had recurrent streptococcal pneumonia in the past. Which one of the following is true regarding her immune system response?

☐ A The innate immune system has produced a streptococcal antigen-specific response
☐ B The innate immune system has led to the activation of phagocytosis
☐ C The innate immune system has activated the classical complement pathway
☐ D The adaptive immune system has led to the release of interferon-α and interferon-β
☐ E The adaptive immune system has responded quickly to release macrophages

33. **Which one of the following statements is true regarding the surface markers of mature T cells?**

☐ A All peripheral blood T cells bear both CD4 and CD8 antigens
☐ B All peripheral blood T cells bear both CD2 and CD3 antigens
☐ C Expression of CD4 allows recognition of MHC class I-associated antigens
☐ D Expression of CD28 is reduced when T-cell activation takes place
☐ E Expression of CD4 occurs mainly in cytotoxic T cells

34. **A five-year-old boy is seen in the Accident and Emergency Department with a history of fever, headache and neck stiffness. A lumbar puncture is performed and the CSF microscopy shows Gram-negative diplococci consistent with *Neisseria meningitidis*. His blood tests reveal a platelet count of 53 × 10⁹/l, a haemoglobin of 12 g/dl and a white cell count (WCC) of 13 × 10⁹/l. He is commenced on intravenous ceftriaxone. On direct questioning of the boy's mother, it appears his past medical history includes recurrent streptococcal respiratory infections and severe eczema. Which rare form of primary immunodeficiency is he most likely to have?**

☐ A Wiskott–Aldrich syndrome
☐ B Job's syndrome
☐ C Chediak–Higashi syndrome
☐ D Bruton's agammaglobulinaemia
☐ E DiGeorge syndrome

35. A 44-year-old geneticist with end-stage renal failure secondary to adult polycystic kidney disease attends the Renal Outpatients Clinic. He has been on haemodialysis for a few years and has had multiple problems with infected fistulae and dialysis catheters. He is awaiting a suitable donor for a renal transplant. He wants to discuss with you the possibility of a porcine implant. Which one of the following is true regarding xenotransplantation?

☐ A Porcine pancreatic islet cell implantation leads to hyperacute rejection
☐ B Acute vascular rejection is the first event after porcine organ transplantation
☐ C Humans naturally possess antibodies to gal-α1,3-gal
☐ D Porcine implants are usually resistant to complement-mediated injury
☐ E Porcine complement regulatory proteins are the same as human ones

36. A 25-year-old Congolese man is admitted via the Accident and Emergency Department with a four-week history of progressive right-sided weakness. Magnetic resonance imaging of his brain reveals changes in the white matter which are consistent with progressive multifocal leukoencephalopathy (PML). After obtaining consent, an HIV test is performed which is positive and T-cell subsets are requested, which reveals a CD4 count of 25 cells/mm^3. Which one of the following immunological techniques was used to ascertain his CD4 count?

☐ A Enzyme-linked immunosorbent assay (ELISA)
☐ B Complement fixation test
☐ C Polymerase chain reaction
☐ D Flow cytometry
☐ E Western blot technique

Answers on pages 93–94

IMMUNOLOGY

Answers

1. **A: Both CD4 and CD8 cells mediate acute rejection following transplantation**

    DRw6-positivity and multiple blood transfusions before surgery have a beneficial effect on outcome following renal transplantation. Matching for major histocompatibility complex (MHC) class II antigens is more important than matching for class I antigens in determining graft survival. Ciclosporin A prevents the activation of T lymphocytes by inhibiting signal transduction within the cytoplasm of T cells. Its major effect is inhibition of interleukin-2 (IL-2) production and thus CD4 cell-dependent proliferative responses; natural killer cell activity is also affected because it depends on IL-2 activity. The drug reduces the incidence of organ rejection and graft-versus-host disease.

2. **E: Non-identical siblings have a 2:4 chance of sharing two antigens**

    The MHC complex is located on the short arm of chromosome 6. Class I antigens are coded for by A, B and C genes, which are present on all nucleated cells and determine graft rejection. Class II antigens are coded for by DP, DQ and DR genes and are present on monocytes/macrophages, B lymphocytes and occasionally on activated T lymphocytes. ABO compatibility (not identical) is essential for transplant viability. The HLA-DR locus is the most important locus governing graft rejection. Non-identical siblings have a 1:4 chance of sharing all four HLA antigens and a 1:4 chance of having no antigens in common.

3. C: It is independent of antibody

Type IV hypersensitivity reactions depend on T lymphocytes, but are independent of antibodies and complement. The incidence of these reactions is usually decreased in HIV infection where there is depletion of CD4 cells. Autoimmune haemolytic anaemia is an example of a type II reaction. Types II and III hypersensitivity are mediated by complement.

	Mechanism	Consequences of hypersensitivity	Disease
Type I (hypersensitvity)	IgE Mast cells Basophils IgG$_4$	Vasodilatation Eosinophils attracted Histamine Leukotrienes, etc	Atopic diseases, eg asthma
Type II (cell-bound antigen)	IgM IgG	Complement activation Cell lysis Opsonisation Neutrophil activation Cell stimulation Blocking Ab	Autoimmune haemolytic anaemia Idiopathic thrombocytopenic purpura Goodpasture's syndrome Pernicious anaemia
Type III (immune complex)	IgG IgA	Circulating immune complexes Complement activation	Serum sickness SLE Henoch–Schönlein purpura Vasculitides Glomerulonephritis
Type IV (delayed)	T cells Macrophaages Antigen-presenting cells	Attraction and activation of lymphocytes and monocytes	TB Graft rejection Graft-versus-host disease Rheumatoid arthritis
Type V	IgG-mediated	Stimulating/blocking cell surface receptors	Graves' disease Myasthenia gravis

4.   D: Hyperthyroidism in Graves' disease

In cell-bound hypersensitivity (type II) circulating antibody (IgG or IgM) binds to cell membrane receptors and activates complement which, in turn, mediates lysis and phagocytosis. Hyperacute rejection is due to preformed circulating cytotoxic antibody which reacts with MHC class I antigens in the donor organ. Graves' disease is an example of type V hypersensitivity (stimulatory) where IgG antibodies (long-acting thyroid stimulator) result in prolonged secretion of thyroid hormone. Another example of type V hypersensitivity occurs in myasthenia gravis.

5.   B: Polyclonal B-cell activation

The major effects of HIV are on T cell-mediated responses. There is a fall in the absolute CD4 cell count and in the CD4:CD8 ratio. There is an associated rise in the number of CD8 suppressor/cytotoxic cells. There is decreased natural killer cell function. The delayed-hypersensitivity skin test, eg the tuberculin test, is impaired as the disease progresses.

6.   A: Soluble CD4 molecules bind to HIV and block its infectivity

The diagnosis of HIV infection is usually confirmed by finding HIV antibody in serum (ELISA). If the ELISA test is positive, then a Western blot assay is usually performed. This process gives a false-positive rate of only 1 in 140,000. The first antibodies to appear are directed against the envelope glycoproteins, gp120 and gp41, which appear three weeks to three months after infection.

7.   D: It is usually IgM

Around 70% of patients with rheumatoid disease have rheumatoid factor in their serum, but a small proportion of patients with moderately active disease are seronegative. Around 5% of the normal population and 20–30% of patients with SLE are rheumatoid factor-positive. The factor itself can be IgM, IgG or IgA. It is directed against the Fc segment of IgG.

8. C: Systemic lupus erythematosus (SLE)

Low complement levels occur in certain diseases and may correlate with disease activity. Examples include post-streptococcal glomerulonephritis, SLE nephritis, membranoproliferative glomerulonephritis, serum sickness, infective endocarditis, disseminated intravascular coagulation, liver disease and septicaemia. In hereditary angioneurotic oedema, there is a hereditary C1 inhibitor deficiency which leads to uncontrolled complement activation.

9. B: T cells make up 70% of circulating lymphocytes

B cells are identified by cell surface immunoglobulin receptors; T cells are identified by rosette formation with sheep red blood cells. T cells comprise 70–80% of the blood lymphocyte population. IgE represents approximately 0.002% of the total immunoglobulin levels in the serum. IgG is the only antibody that can cross the placenta.

10. D: Malaria

Acquired hypogammaglobulinaemia may be due to one of the following mechanisms:

1. Decreased production – severe malnutrition, lymphoproliferative disease, infection (malaria, septicaemia, trypanasomiasis), drugs (eg cytotoxic agents, gold, phenytoin, penicillamine), irradiation, splenectomy
2. Increased loss or catabolism – protein-losing enteropathy and intestinal lymphangiectasia, malabsorption, nephrotic syndrome, exfoliative dermatitis, burns.

Polyclonal hypergammaglobulinaemia can occur in chronic infections (eg tuberculosis, leishmaniasis, infective endocarditis), autoimmune diseases (SLE, rheumatoid arthritis), ulcerative colitis and Crohn's disease, sarcoidosis and hepatic disease.

11. B: Polyarteritis nodosa

Antinuclear antibodies (ANAs) are IgM or IgG antibodies directed against a variety of nuclear constituents (eg DNA or RNA). High titres are seen in SLE, other connective tissue diseases (eg rheumatoid arthritis, systemic sclerosis, Sjögren's syndrome), autoimmune diseases (eg myasthenia gravis, chronic active hepatitis), and with the use of certain drugs (eg drug-induced SLE syndrome). There are four ANA staining patterns:

Pattern	Disease association	Antigen
Homogeneous	Common pattern	DNA histone
Speckled	SLE, Sjögren's syndrome Mixed connective tissue disorder	Extractable nuclear antigen
Nucleolar	Scleroderma, SLE	Nucleolar DNA
Centromere	CREST syndrome Diffuse scleroderma	Centromere

12. C: Post-streptococcal glomerulonephritis

There are three different mechanisms which are responsible for diseases resulting from the formation of immune complexes:

1. The combined effects of a low-grade, persistent infection (eg infection with α-haemolytic *Streptococcus viridans* or *Plasmodium vivax*, or viral hepatitis), together with a weak antibody response.
2. The continued production of antibody to self-antigen, leading to prolonged immune complex formation, eg SLE, rheumatoid arthritis, polyarteritis, polymyositis/dermatomyositis, cutaneous vasculitis, cryoglobulinaemia and fibrosing alveolitis.
3. Formation of immune complexes at body surfaces, especially in the lungs, following repeated inhalation of antigenic material from moulds, plants or animals, eg pigeon fancier's lung and farmer's lung.

13. **E: Scleroderma**

   The delayed hypersensitivity reaction is an immune function test which measures the presence of activated T cells that recognise a certain substance. Delayed hypersensitivity reactions are impaired in patients with sarcoidosis, malignant lymphomas or the DiGeorge syndrome, and in those receiving corticosteroid therapy. Impaired delayed hypersensitivity increases susceptibility to opportunistic infections and severe viral infections and immunisation with live vaccines may cause fatal generalised reactions. The Wiscott–Aldrich syndrome is a combined B- and T-cell disorder with an X-linked inheritance. Immunological changes in malnutrition include loss of delayed hypersensitivity, fewer T lymphocytes, impaired lymphocyte response and decreased secretory immunoglobulin A (IgA).

14. **B: It is the predominant cause of shock in Gram-negative septicaemia**

   Tumor necrosis factor (TNF) is a cytokine released by macrophages/monocytes. It is the principal mediator of the host response to Gram-negative bacteria, but may also play a role in the response to other infectious organisms. It activates inflammatory leucocytes to kill microbes, stimulates mononuclear phagocytes to produce cytokines, acts as a co-stimulator for T-cell activation and antibody production by B cells, and exerts an interferon-like effect against viruses. It enhances the microbicidal capacity of macrophages and neutrophils, causes NK cells to release interferon-γ, and causes changes in endothelial cells, increasing the entry of cells into sites of inflammation.

15. **C: A Mantoux-positive schoolchild**

   BCG should be given to unvaccinated healthcare workers, any unvaccinated contact with active TB, immigrants from areas with a high prevalence of TB and their children, and to neonates born into a family where there is active TB. BCG is contraindicated in immunosuppressed patients.

16. **A: It has a key role in mucosal immunity**

IgA is the main immunoglobulin in secretions of the respiratory and gastrointestinal tract, and in sweat, saliva, tears and colostrum, and it has a key defence role for mucosal surfaces. It polymerises to a dimer intracellularly by binding through a cysteine-rich polypeptide JC chain synthesised locally by mucosal cells. When aggregated, it binds polymorphs and activates complement by the alternative pathway.

17. **D: They include the slow-reacting substance of anaphylaxis (SRS-A)**

Leukotrienes are made by eosinophils, basophils and mast cells and are mediators of inflammation and allergic reactions. They cause arteriolar constriction and bronchoconstriction, increase vascular permeability and attract neutrophils and eosinophils to the site of inflammation. Leukotriene D4 (LTD4) is SRS-A, which causes smooth muscle contraction. Montelukast inhibits the action of LTD4 at its receptor. Prostaglandins, prostacyclins, thromboxanes and leukotrienes are derived from arachidonic acid via the cyclooxygenase and lipoxygenase pathways.

18. **D: It is stimulated by cytokines**

The acute phase proteins include proteins which act as mediators (as in opsonisation – C3 and C4 complement components, C-reactive protein), enzyme inhibitors (α_1-antitrypsin) and scavengers (haptoglobin). Inflammation activates macrophages and lymphocytes to produce cytokines (particularly interleukin-6) which stimulate the production of acute phase proteins by the liver. C-reactive protein is used to measure the acute phase response. C peptide is produced in the pancreas during the manufacture of insulin. There is only a minor acute phase response in viral infections compared with bacterial infections. An acute phase response may occur in inflammatory conditions, after trauma, post-operatively, associated with malignancy, or in autoimmune disease.

19. E: Wegener's granulomatosis

Cytoplasmic-staining antineutrophil cytoplasmic antibody
(c-ANCA) is present in 95% of patients with active generalised
Wegener's granulomatosis. Perinuclear-staining ANCA (p-ANCA)
is classically associated with microscopic polyangiitis but may also
be found in SLE, mixed connective tissue disorder, chronic active
hepatitis and other autoimmune disease. ANCA-associated
glomerulonephritis is now the most commonly recognised form of
rapidly progressive glomerulonephritis.

20. C: Isolated IgA deficiency

In isolated IgA deficiency, where IgG levels are normal or elevated,
intravenous immunoglobulin treatment is contraindicated. Such
patients may have anti-IgA antibodies, resulting in anaphylactic
shock if the administered gamma globulin contains IgA. There is no
effective replacement therapy for IgA.

21. D: It is responsible for the determination of blood group

IgM antibody is mainly intravascular. It is made up of five
monomeric subunits. It activates complement via the classical
pathway and it does not cross the placenta. It is the principal
immunoglobulin of the primary immune response. The serum
concentration of IgM is characteristically reduced in patients with
uncontrolled coeliac disease. Its levels may return to normal
with a gluten-free diet. The half-life of IgM is approximately five
days.

22. C: Meningoencephalitis due to echovirus infection

Bruton's agammaglobulinaemia is a rare X-linked inherited
disorder which presents in male infants with recurrent pyogenic
and gastrointestinal infections at around six months of age. There is
an absence of circulating B cells but T cells are normal or increased
in number. Infections with *Staphylococcus, Streptococcus* and
Haemophilus are common but these patients are also susceptible to
enteroviruses such as echoviruses. Recurrent sinopulmonary

infections are characteristic. The defective gene (tyrosine-kinase mutation) on the X chromosome has been identified. The condition usually presents with recurrent respiratory tract infections between six and 18 months of age. Tonsils and palpable lymphoid tissue may be absent. Mucocutaneous candidiasis usally occurs with T cell dysfunction and aspergillosis is more prominent in inherited neutrophil disorders.

23.   **B: They act within infected cells to inhibit virus replication**

Interferons (IFNs) are glycoproteins produced by virus-infected cells. Properties include prevention of viral replication, anti-tumour activity, and the activation of macrophages and natural killer cells. IFN-α and IFN-β lead to enhanced MHC class I expression, whereas IFN-γ leads to both MHC class I and MHC class II expression. IFN-γ also mediates suppression of T_H2 cells. Tumour necrosis factor-α (TFN-α) is the principal mediator in the host response to Gram-negative bacterial infection.

24.   **E: The prolonged clotting time does not correct with normal plasma**

In primary antiphospholipid antibody (APA) syndrome the antibody titre is high. The classic presentation is of vascular thrombosis and recurrent fetal loss. The frequency of different presentations is as follows:

Deep vein thrombosis	54%
Arterial thrombosis	44%
Recurrent fetal loss	34%
Pulmonary embolism	18%
Cerebrovascular accident	13%

These patients should be anticoagulated for life. The syndrome is associated with a false-positive VDRL. Antibodies to dsDNA are not found in patients with APA syndrome. There is considerable overlap in the clinical features associated with antiphospholipid antibodies and with lupus anticoagulant. Common to both SLE and the APA syndrome is failure of the clotting defect to correct with normal plasma, which implies that an antibody is present.

	SLE	APA syndrome
Gender, female:male	9:1	2:1
Mean age, years	24	38
Antinuclear antibody, %	>90	45
Antibodies to dsDNA, %	80	0
Antiphospholipid antibodies,%	40	100

25. E: *Trypanosoma brucei*

Antigenic variation is best recognised in the organisms causing trypanosomiasis and influenza, but also in some bacteria, such as meningococci. After infection with *Trypanosoma brucei,* destruction of trypanosomes by host antibody is followed by the emergence of parasites expressing different surface antigens, or variant surface glycoproteins. This type of antigenic variation is known as 'phenotypic variation', in contrast to genotypic variation, in which a new strain periodically results in an epidemic (eg influenza virus epidemics).

26. C: It is useful in the treatment of chronic granulomatous disease

Interferon-γ (IFN-γ) is released by human T lymphocytes and has an antiviral action via activation of natural killer cells, up-regulation of MHC class I and II antigens on virally infected cells, and inhibition of viral replication. Genetically engineered recombinant IFN-α, IFN-β and IFN-γ are all available but IFN-α has been the most extensively studied. It has a role in the management of poorly responsive malignancies, such as hairy cell leukaemia and renal cell carcinoma. It is also useful as an antiviral agent, producing significant clearance of hepatitis B in chronic carriers and histological improvement in 50% of patients with hepatitis C. IFN-γ has been shown to be useful in the management of chronic granulomatous diseases, a group of inherited conditions resulting in recurrent pyogenic infections.

27. **B: Production of IgE**

CD4 T cells can be divided into different subsets depending on their cytokine profile. CD4 cells that produce IL-2 and IFN-γ, but not IL-4, are designated 'T_H1' and are chiefly responsible for delayed-type hypersensitivity reactions. In contrast, CD4 T cells that produce IL-4 and IL-5, but not IL-2 and IFN-γ, are designated 'T_H2'. They are efficient helper cells for antibody production, especially IgE and IgG$_1$.

28. **A: They are found in nearly all patients with primary biliary cirrhosis**

Over 95% of patients with primary biliary cirrhosis (PBC) have circulating antimitochondrial antibodies; the absence of the antibodies virtually excludes the diagnosis. They are also found in a small proportion of patients with chronic active hepatitis (CAH) and cryptogenic cirrhosis. The cause of the bile duct damage seen in PBC is unclear, but it may be mediated by cytotoxic T cells. Unlike CAH, PBC is not associated with any particular HLA antigens. IgM is raised in >80% of patients with PBC; IgG is elevated in CAH.

29. **D: They act as receptors for the presentation of antigen to helper T cells**

Class II MHC molecules have a restricted distribution compared with class I molecules, which are found on all nucleated cells. Class II molecules are normally found on B lymphocytes, activated T cells, macrophages and inflamed vascular endothelium. Human histocompatibility antigens are remarkable for their degree of polymorphism, meaning that the genetic variability between individuals is very great and most unrelated individuals possess different HLA molecules. Antigen processing is crucial for the recognition of antigen by T cells. Processed antigen is presented to T cells alongside the MHC class II antigens on the surface of specialised cells known as 'antigen-presenting cells' (APCs). T cells do not recognise processed antigen alone: CD4 helper T cells recognise antigen with class II molecules; and CD8 suppressor/

cytotoxic T cells recognise antigens with MHC class I molecules. Class I antigens determine graft rejection.

30. **C: Follicular dendritic cells**

Antigen-presenting cells (APCs) are a heterogeneous population of lymphocytes that are found primarily in the skin, lymph nodes, spleen and thymus. They may have a pivotal role in the induction of the functional activity of helper T cells, or may communicate with other leucocytes. The classic APCs are the Langerhans cells in the skin and the follicular dendritic cells, which are found in the secondary follicles of the B-cell areas of the lymph nodes and spleen. The Langerhans cells are rich in class II MHC molecules for communicating with CD4 and T cells, whereas follicular dendritic cells do not express class II MHC molecules. B cells and macrophages are also efficient antigen-presenting cells.

31. **D: SLE – deposits of immunoglobulin and complement along the basement membrane zone**

Pemphigoid is characterised by autoantibodies to the basement membrane layer. Pemphigus is associated with autoantibodies to epidermal intracelluar cement, and dermatitis herpetiformis with coarse granular deposits of IgA in dermal papillae. In bullous skin eruptions, direct immunofluorescence of peri-lesional skin rather than of established bullae is diagnostic.

32. **B: The innate immune system has led to the activation of phagocytosis**

The innate immune system is the body's first line of attack and responds rapidly (within minutes) to infection. It fights general classes of pathogens with the same molecules and cells (unlike the adaptive immune system which produces an antigen-specific response). The innate immune system stimulates phagocytosis by macrophages and neutrophil granulocytes and activates the alternative complement pathway (C1-5 and C6-9, leading to the formation of the membrane attack complex). Interferon-α and

IMMUNOLOGY – ANSWERS

interferon-β are important in viral resistance. The adaptive immune system responds slowly over days to weeks via humoral and cell-mediated responses.

33 **B: All peripheral blood T cells bear both CD2 and CD3 antigens**

All mature thymocytes and peripheral blood T cells bear the CD2, CD3, CD5, and CD28 antigens. T cells are divided into CD4 and CD8 subsets and CD4+ cells are further subdivided into T_H1 and T_H2 cells on the basis of their cytokine profiles. Cytotoxic T cells (T_C) express mainly CD8, and lyse autologous cells bearing foreign antigen molecules associated with MHC class I, whereas CD4 T cells recognise antigen associated with MHC class II molecules. CD28 is present in the highest amount in activated T cells. It is a T-cell co-stimulatory molecule that plays a major role in T-cell activation.

34 **A: Wiskott–Aldrich syndrome**

Wiskott–Aldrich syndrome is a rare, X-linked recessive, combined B- and T-cell disorder. It has an incidence of approximately four per million male births. It usually presents with severe eczema, thrombocytopenia and recurrent pyogenic infections (eg *Streptococcus pneumoniae, Neisseria meningitidis, Haemophilus influenzae*). There is an increased incidence of lymphoreticular system tumours and low IgM levels are found in the presence of increased IgE levels. Bruton's agammaglobulinaemia is an X-linked recessive B-cell disorder. DiGeorge syndrome is non-familial and characterised by congenital thymic aplasia, cardiovascular defects, hypoparathyroidism, seizures and opportunistic infections. Chediak–Higashi syndrome and Job's syndrome are neutrophil disorders.

35 **C: Humans naturally possess antibodies to gal-α1,3-gal**

Hyperacute rejection can occur in any transplanted organ (human or animal) within minutes to hours. It is characterised by platelet aggregation and interstitial haemorrhage in the transplanted organ.

93

It is not seen in transplanted cells (eg pancreatic islet cell transplantation). Hyperacute rejection in porcine implants is mediated by two factors:

1. All lower mammals express a sugar called 'gal-α1,3-gal', which is not found in humans, apes or old-world monkeys. All humans posses natural antibodies against gal-α1,3-gal.
2. There is profound activation of the complement cascade, leading to extensive complement-mediated injury in the transplanted organ. The xenograft is very susceptible to this as porcine complement regulatory proteins cannot dampen the response well.

36   D: Flow cytometry

Flow cytometry is a technique used to detect cell surface antigens (eg CD4) and cell markers in haematological malignancy. Blood cells are mixed with fluorochrome-labelled monoclonal antibodies that bind to cell surface markers. The flow cytometer then detects fluorescence and counts the number of cells bound by monoclonal antibodies. It can also be used to measure cell properties such as cell viability, proliferation and intracellular enzyme activity.

Chapter 5
ANATOMY
Questions

1. **Which one of the following is true regarding the subclavian artery?**

   - [ ] A It becomes the axillary artery at the medial border of the first rib
   - [ ] B It passes deep to scalenus anterior
   - [ ] C It arises from the aortic arch on the right side
   - [ ] D It arises from the brachiocephalic trunk on the left side
   - [ ] E It gives off the posterior intercostal arteries

2. **Which one of the following is the correct pairing of reflex and innervating spinal segment?**

   - [ ] A Ankle jerk – S1
   - [ ] B Knee jerk – L1/L2
   - [ ] C Biceps jerk – C7/C8
   - [ ] D Triceps jerk – T1
   - [ ] E Cremasteric reflex – S2/S3

3. **Which one of the following is true regarding the left main bronchus?**

   - [ ] A It is shorter than the right main bronchus
   - [ ] B It passes posterior to the oesophagus
   - [ ] C It contains complete rings of cartilage
   - [ ] D It divides into three secondary bronchi
   - [ ] E It divides into ten tertiary bronchi

Answers on page 107

4. A 76-year-old man underwent a transurethral resection of the prostate gland for benign prostatic hyperplasia. During this procedure he was kept in the lithotomy position for two hours and sustained a compression injury to the femoral nerve. Which one of the following neurological findings will be present?

- [ ] A Failure of adduction of the thigh at the hip joint
- [ ] B Sensory loss over the medial aspect of the lower leg
- [ ] C Foot drop
- [ ] D Paraesthesia of the lateral aspect of the foot
- [ ] E Failure of knee flexion

5. A 45-year-old woman with rheumatoid arthritis presents with a one-week history of a flare-up of pain and swelling involving her wrists. Clinical assessment and radiology reveal the presence of a synovial cyst overlying and compressing the ulnar nerve in the wrist. Which one of the following findings will be present?

- [ ] A Wasting of the thenar eminence
- [ ] B Loss of sensation over the medial one and a half fingers
- [ ] C Loss of the pincer action of the thumb and forefinger
- [ ] D Wrist drop
- [ ] E Wasting of the first and second lumbricals

6. Which one of the following is true of the abdominal aorta?

- [ ] A It passes through the diaphragm at the level of T10
- [ ] B It is closely related to the right sympathetic trunk
- [ ] C It gives off four lumbar arteries on each side
- [ ] D Aneurysms are usually suprarenal
- [ ] E It divides into the common iliac arteries at the level of L2

7. **Which one of the the following statements is true regarding the thoracic duct?**

☐ A It enters the thorax to the right of the oesophagus
☐ B It ascends first behind and then to the left of the aorta
☐ C It passes behind the first part of the subclavian artery
☐ D It terminates at the union of the superior vena cava and the brachiocephalic veins
☐ E It drains the entire lymphatic field below the diaphragm and the right half of the field above it

8. **Which one of the following is true of the median nerve?**

☐ A It derives its fibres from spinal segments C6–8 and T1
☐ B It gives off a branch to innervate the triceps muscle
☐ C It supplies the ulnar half of flexor digitorum profundus
☐ D Damage to it at the wrist causes wasting of the hypothenar muscles
☐ E It gives off sensory branches to the dorsal aspect of the lateral two and a half fingers

9. **Which one of the following pairings of muscle/muscle action and innervating nerve(s) is correct?**

☐ A Quadriceps – sciatic nerve (S1/S2)
☐ B Splaying of the fingers – median nerve (C8)
☐ C Main supinator of the forearm – deep branch of the radial nerve (C7/C8)
☐ D Extensors of the hand at the wrist joint – deep branch of the radial nerve (C8)
☐ E Ankle dorsiflexion – tibial nerve (S1/S2)

10. **Which one of the following pairings of cutaneous area and sensory root is correct?**

☐ A The sole of the foot – S3
☐ B The little finger – C6
☐ C The groin – L5
☐ D The index finger – C7
☐ E The umbilicus – T10

11. **Which one of the following statements about the spinal cord is correct?**

☐ A The subdural space contains the cerebrospinal fluid (CSF)
☐ B The T12 segment lies at the level of the T11 vertebral body
☐ C Hemisection results in contralateral loss of pain and temperature sensation below the level of the lesion
☐ D It transmits two-point discrimination sensation in the lateral spinothalamic tract
☐ E The anterior spinal arteries supply the whole cord

12. **A 54-year-old man is referred by his general practitioner with a two-month history of tiredness. A full blood count shows a haemoglobin level of 6.4 g/dl. He gives a history of heavy alcohol consumption over many years. An ultrasound scan of his liver shows cirrhosis with portal hypertension. Persistent minor blood loss from varices is suspected. In which one of the following sites may a portosystemic anastomosis be present?**

☐ A The middle third of the oesophagus
☐ B The first part of the duodenum
☐ C The splenic bed
☐ D Along the falciform ligament
☐ E The superior rectal wall

13. Which one of the following is a feature of an injury to the common peroneal nerve?

   ☐ A Equinovarus deformity of the foot
   ☐ B Loss of sensation in the sole of the foot
   ☐ C Calcaneovalgus deformity of the foot
   ☐ D Positive Trendelenburg test
   ☐ E Claw-like deformity of the toes

14. A 40-year-old woman attends her general practitioner because she has noticed drooping of the left side of her mouth. She has no other symptoms. Examination of the cranial nerves reveals a lower motor neurone lesion of the left facial nerve, and no other abnormality. The general practitioner diagnoses Bell's palsy and reassures the patient.Which one of the following statements about the facial nerve is true?

   ☐ A It supplies taste to the posterior two-thirds of the tongue
   ☐ B It leaves the skull via the foramen ovale
   ☐ C Injury to the nerve at a supranuclear level causes paralysis of the forehead muscles
   ☐ D It carries fibres in the corneal reflex
   ☐ E Section of the nerve in the auditory canal causes ipsilateral hypersecretion of tears

15. A nurse presents to Casualty complaining of severe back pain and inability to walk, which has been getting progressively worse over the last three weeks. Urgent magnetic resonance imaging (MRI) confirms a prolapsed intervertebral disc affecting the S1 root. Which one of the following findings will be present?

   ☐ A A positive femoral stretch test
   ☐ B Impaired knee jerk
   ☐ C Paraesthesia on the medial aspect of the foot
   ☐ D Weakness of dorsiflexion of the foot
   ☐ E Limitation of straight leg raising

Answers on pages 109–111

16. **Which one of the following statements about the oesophagus is true?**

- ☐ A It runs from the upper border of the cricoid cartilage
- ☐ B It is crossed by the right main bronchus
- ☐ C It leaves the thorax at the level of T10
- ☐ D Portosystemic anastamosis usually occurs in the middle third
- ☐ E The squamo-epithelial junction is the commonest site for the development of carcinoma

17. **Which one of the following is true of the radial nerve?**

- ☐ A Injury at the elbow results in loss of pronation of the forearm
- ☐ B It derives its fibres from the C6–8 and T1 roots of the brachial plexus
- ☐ C It gives off a branch to the biceps muscle
- ☐ D Section of the nerve will cause loss of sensation in the tip of the middle finger
- ☐ E Damage in the axilla will cause atrophy of triceps

18. **A 45-year-old man is admitted to the Intensive Care Unit in severe septic shock. Central venous cannulation of the internal jugular vein is required for ongoing haemodynamic monitoring.Which one of the following is true regarding the internal jugular vein?**

- ☐ A It originates at the foramen magnum
- ☐ B It passes behind the thoracic duct on the left side
- ☐ C It lies medial to the common carotid artery, outside the carotid sheath
- ☐ D It contains valves in dilated segments at its superior and inferior ends
- ☐ E It joins the superior vena cava at the lower border of the first costal cartilage

19. **A 22-year-old woman presents with a painless midline swelling in the upper third of her neck. The lump moves on protrusion of the tongue and the patient is clinically and biochemically euthyroid. Which one of the following statements is true regarding the thyroid gland?**

- [ ] A   The isthmus overlies the third to the sixth rings of the trachea
- [ ] B   Follicular cells arise from the epithelium of the dorsal wing of the fourth pharyngeal pouch
- [ ] C   The thyroglossal tract arises at the junction of the anterior third and the posterior two-thirds of the tongue
- [ ] D   Approximately 50% of thyroglossal cysts are found lateral to the midline
- [ ] E   A thyroglossal fistula usually arises as a result of rupture of a thyroglossal cyst

20. **Which one of the following is true of the inferior vena cava (IVC)?**

- [ ] A   It joins the superior vena cava 4 cm above the right atrium
- [ ] B   It runs to the left of the aorta
- [ ] C   It receives the two hepatic veins
- [ ] D   It is formed by the two common iliac veins anterior to the right common iliac artery
- [ ] E   It receives the left suprarenal vein directly

21. **Which one of these clinical signs results from injury of the T1 root of the brachial plexus?**

- [ ] A   Wrist drop
- [ ] B   Loss of elbow flexion
- [ ] C   Loss of cutaneous sensation over the lateral two fingers
- [ ] D   Horner's syndrome
- [ ] E   An Erb–Duchenne palsy

22. **Which one of the following muscles assists in the inversion of the foot?**

- A Tibialis posterior
- B Flexor hallucis longus
- C Extensor digitorum longus
- D Peroneus longus
- E Gastrocnemius

23. **An 80-year-old woman with a history of hypertension and peripheral vascular disease attends her local optician, complaining of 'problems with her eyes'. The optician refers her for an urgent ophthalmological assessment. Clinical examination and perimetry show a left homonymous hemianopia. Computed tomography (CT) will reveal a lesion of which one of these structures?**

- A Optic chiasm
- B Right optic radiation
- C Left optic nerve
- D Left optic tract
- E Right optic tract

24. **Which one of the following neurological problems is caused by the accompanying vascular insult?**

- A Left-sided face and arm weakness – right anterior cerebral artery occlusion
- B Right-sided neglect – left posterior cerebral artery occlusion
- C Right homonymous hemianopia – left middle cerebral artery occlusion
- D Akinetic mute state – left anterior cerebral artery occlusion
- E Right-sided Horner's syndrome – right anterior inferior cerebellar artery

25. **Which one of the following results from injury to the corticospinal pathway on the left side at C2?**

    ☐ A Weakness of limb muscles on the right side
    ☐ B Brisk reflexes on the right side
    ☐ C Spasticity of muscles on the left side
    ☐ D Fasciculation of the muscles on the left side
    ☐ E Up-going plantar on the right side

26. **Which one of the following is true of the trochlear nerve?**

    ☐ A It supplies the superior rectus muscle
    ☐ B It decussates before leaving the brainstem
    ☐ C It runs along the medial wall of the cavernous sinus
    ☐ D A lesion causes a divergent squint
    ☐ E Damage is most commonly due to head injury

27. **A 70-year-old man, who is known to have hormone-resistant carcinoma of the prostate, is brought into hospital by ambulance, having 'gone off his legs'. He relates that he has been suffering from severe pain affecting his back and chest wall, and that he has been incontinent for five days. Magnetic resonance imaging shows a metastatic tumour deposit completely obliterating his spinal cord at the level of T6. Which one of the following would be characteristic of this spinal cord lesion?**

    ☐ A Permanent loss of tendon reflexes in the lower limbs
    ☐ B Impotence
    ☐ C Return of voluntary sphincter control
    ☐ D Permanent loss of voluntary control of the limb muscles
    ☐ E Transient loss of sensation below the level of the lesion

28. A 22-year-old medical student presents to his general practitioner with sensory disturbance and weakness affecting his left arm. He gives a vague history of occasional pains affecting his whole arm, but cannot recall experiencing any minor trauma. On examination, there is sensory loss, predominantly affecting the middle finger. There is weakness of forearm extension as well as wrist flexion and extension. The triceps reflex is absent. Which one of the following would explain this pattern of neurological loss?

☐ A Compression of C7/C8/T1 due to cervical spondylosis
☐ B Compression of C7 secondary to disc herniation
☐ C Compression of T1 fibres secondary to neurogenic thoracic outlet syndrome
☐ D Injury to the radial nerve secondary to prolonged pressure ('Saturday night palsy')
☐ E Injury to the ulnar nerve at the elbow secondary to entrapment

29. A 76-year-old man is admitted to hospital with dizziness and chest pain. An ECG reveals Mobitz type II second-degree heart block at the rate of 46 beats per minute. While waiting for the medical registrar to arrive, he is given a total of 3 mg of atropine with little effect and goes on to require temporary cardiac pacing. Which one of the following side effects might he experience as a result of this drug therapy?

☐ A Bronchoconstriction
☐ B Urinary incontinence
☐ C Increased lacrimation
☐ D Constipation
☐ E Mild sedation

30. A 67-year-old woman is admitted to the Coronary Care Unit with acute shortness of breath secondary to pulmonary oedema. She is managed with intravenous furosemide (frusemide), an intravenous nitrate infusion and continuous positive airways pressure (CPAP) ventilatory support. She continues to deteriorate, with a PO_2 of 5.7 kPa, a pH of 7.14 and a minimal urine output. She is in sinus rhythm at a rate of 92 beats per minute and has a blood pressure of 120/76 mmHg. The cardiology registrar on call suggests commencing inotropic/vasopressive therapy. Which one of the following drugs would be the most appropriate choice?

- [ ] A Adrenaline (epinephrine)
- [ ] B Noradrenaline (norepinephrine)
- [ ] C Phenylephrine
- [ ] D Renal-dose dopamine
- [ ] E Dobutamine

31. A 65-year-old alcoholic man presents to hospital with confusion, nystagmus and ataxia. A diagnosis of Wernicke's encephalopathy is made and the patient is treated with intravenous Pabrinex®. The neurological features resolve over the next few days, but it becomes evident that he has severe anterograde and retrograde amnesia. Long-term memory is well preserved. Which one of these areas of the brain is likely to have been damaged?

- [ ] A Amygdala
- [ ] B Mamillary bodies
- [ ] C Hippocampus
- [ ] D Hypothalamus
- [ ] E Cingulate gyrus

32. A 78-year-old man is admitted to the Accident and Emergency
Department feeling unwell and complaining of sensory
disturbance. He has a history of hypertension and diabetes
mellitus and is known to have prostatic carcinoma with bony
metastases. On examination of the peripheral nervous system, the
medical senior house officer finds loss of pinprick and
temperature sensation on in the right arm and leg with no
associated right-sided weakness.Which one of the following
would best explain the neurological findings?

- A   Right-sided Brown–Séquard syndrome
- B   Left-sided lateral medullary syndrome
- C   Left-sided thalamic infarct
- D   Right-sided thalamic infarct
- E   Left middle cerebral artery occlusion

Answer on page 115

ANATOMY

Answers

---

1. B: It passes deep to scalenus anterior

The subclavian artery arises from the aortic arch on the left, and the brachiocephalic trunk on the right. It runs deep to the scalenus anterior muscle and becomes the axillary artery at the lateral border of the first rib. Its branches include the vertebral, internal thoracic, deep cervical and high intercostal arteries, and the thyrocervical trunk.

2. A: Ankle jerk – S1

The ankle jerk is mediated by the tibial branch of the sciatic nerve. The knee jerk is innervated by the femoral nerve (L3/L4); the biceps jerk originates from C5 and C6 (the musculocutaneous nerve); the triceps jerk is controlled by the radial nerve (C7); and the cremasteric reflex is innervated by L1 and L2.

3. E: It divides into ten tertiary bronchi

The left main bronchus is longer than the right main bronchus and its angle is more acute. It passes anterior to the oesophagus and the descending aorta and reaches the hilum of the lung at the level of T6. It divides into two main bronchi, the upper lobe bronchus (which gives off the lingular lobe bronchus) and the lower lobe bronchus. These then divide into a total of ten tertiary bronchi. The walls of the left main bronchus contain C-shaped cartilage rings; only the trachea has complete rings.

4. **B: Sensory loss over the medial aspect of the lower leg**

The femoral nerve arises from L3 and L4. It supplies the muscles of the anterolateral thigh, the quadriceps muscle (which effects knee extension) and sartorius. Its sensory branches innervate the medial aspect of the lower leg and foot and the anteromedial aspect of the thigh. Hip adduction is mainly supplied by the obturator nerve. A common peroneal nerve lesion would cause foot drop and paraesthesia of the lateral side of the foot.

5. **B: Loss of sensation over the medial one and a half fingers**

Damage to the ulnar nerve at the wrist results in a claw hand. This is due to wasting and paralysis of the hypothenar muscles and the intrinsic small muscles of the hand. The lateral two lumbricals are spared as these, along with the thenar eminence, are innervated by the median nerve. The ulnar nerve supplies sensation to the medial one and a half fingers and the adjacent palmar and dorsal surfaces of the hand.

6. **C: It gives off four lumbar arteries on each side**

The aorta enters the abdomen after piercing the diaphragm at the T12 level. Through its course in the abdomen it is closely related to the left sympathetic trunk. It divides into the common iliac arteries at the level of L4. Aneurysms are infrarenal in 95% of cases and are usually atherosclerotic in origin.

7. **C: It passes behind the first part of the subclavian artery**

The thoracic duct drains the entire lymphatic field below the diaphragm and the left half of the field above it. It begins at the cisterna chyli and enters the thorax on the right side of the aorta. It ascends first behind and then to the left of the oesophagus. It passes behind the carotid sheath at the level of C7 and behind the subclavian artery. It empties into the venous system at the junction of the left subclavian and internal jugular veins.

8. **A: It derives its fibres from spinal segments C6–8 and T1**

   The median nerve arises from the lateral and medial cords of the brachial plexus (C6–8, T1). It gives off no branches in the arm. It supplies the radial half of the flexor digitorum profundus (the ulnar nerve supplies the ulnar half), the first (lateral) two lumbricals, the thenar eminence muscles and sensation to the lateral three and a half fingers.

9. **D: Extensors of the hand at the wrist joint – deep branch of the radial nerve (C8)**

   Quadriceps is innervated by the femoral nerve (L3/L4). Splaying of the fingers is performed by the small muscles of the hand supplied by the ulnar nerve (T1). The main supinator of the forearm is biceps brachialis and this is innervated by the musculocutaneous nerve (C5/C6). The anterior tibial muscles perform dorsiflexion of the ankle and are supplied by the peroneal nerve (L4/L5).

10. **E: The umbilicus – T10**

    The sole of the foot is innervated by S1, the groin by L1, the index finger by C6, the middle finger by C7 and the little finger by C8.

11. **C: Hemisection results in contralateral loss of pain and temperature sensation below the level of the lesion**

    The CSF is contained in the subarachnoid space. Hemisection of the cord results in ipsilateral paralysis and contralateral loss of pain and temperature sensation (the Brown–Séquard syndrome). Two-point discrimination sensations are carried in the posterior columns. The anterior spinal arteries supply the anterior two-thirds of the cord. The remainder is supplied by the posterior arteries, which are branches of the vertebral arteries or of the posterior inferior cerebellar arteries.

12. **D: Along the falciform ligament**

There are several areas of communication between the portal and systemic venous systems. The oesophageal branches of the left gastric vein and the oesophageal veins of the azygous system communicate around the lower third of the oesophagus and the cardia of the stomach. The inferior haemorrhoidal veins join the inferior mesenteric vein of the portal system. There are portal tributaries in the mesentery, mesocolon and retroperitoneum which communicate with the renal, phrenic and portal veins. Veins of the anterior abdominal wall which pass to the umbilicus along the falciform ligament join portal branches in the liver. Portal branches of the liver also communicate with the veins of the diaphragm across the bare area of the liver.

13. **A: Equinovarus deformity of the foot**

The common peroneal nerve supplies the muscles of the anterior compartment of the leg. These act to turn the leg upwards and outwards. Its sensory supply is to the anterolateral aspect of the foot, including the dorsum of the ankle. Injury to the common peroneal nerve causes foot drop, with loss of dorsiflexion and foot eversion and paralysis of toe extension, leading to an equinovarus deformity of the foot. Claw-like deformity of the toes, loss of sensation in the sole of the foot and a calcaneovalgus deformity are features of a tibial nerve injury.

14. **D: It carries fibres in the corneal reflex**

The facial nerve supplies taste fibres to the anterior two-thirds of the tongue. It leaves the skull through the stylomastoid foramen. A supranuclear lesion of the nerve spares the forehead muscles, which receive bilateral cortical fibres. The facial nerve carries fibres in the efferent arc of the corneal reflex, supplying orbicularis oculi. Section of the nerve in the auditory canal will cause loss of tear secretion in the ipsilateral eye.

15. E: Limitation of straight leg raising

In S1 root lesions, there is weakness of the plantar flexors of the foot, impairment of the ankle jerk and paraesthesia over the lateral aspect of the foot.

16. C: It leaves the thorax at the level of T10

The oesophagus runs from the lower border of the cricoid cartilage (C6) and leaves the thorax at the level of T10. The lower third of the oesophagus is drained by the portal venous system via the gastric veins. Around 50% of oesophageal carcinomas occur in the middle third and 25% in the lower third of the oesophagus. Distal tumours are more likely to be adenocarcinoma.

17. E: Damage in the axilla will cause atrophy of triceps

The radial nerve arises from the main branch of the posterior cord of the brachial plexus (C5–8). It supplies the extensor muscles of the upper limb. Injury to the radial nerve in the axilla causes wrist drop, atrophy of triceps and paraesthesia of the dorsum of the hand between the first and second metacarpals. Biceps is innervated by the musculocutaneous nerve. Damage to the median nerve at the elbow will cause loss of pronation.

18. D: It contains valves in dilated segments at its superior and inferior ends

The internal jugular vein drains the cranial cavity and some of the superficial veins of the head and neck. It contains valves in dilated segments at its superior and inferior ends (bulbs). It orginates in the jugular foramen and descends within the carotid sheath, lying lateral first to the internal carotid artery and then to the common carotid artery. It passes anterior to the thoracic duct on the left side. It joins the subclavian vein to form the brachiocephalic trunk.

19. E: A thyroglossal fistula usually arises as a result of rupture of a thyroglossal cyst

Thyroid follicular cells arise from epithelial proliferation at the base of the pharynx. The thyroglossal tract arises from the foramen caecum, at the junction of the anterior two-thirds and the posteior third of the tongue. The isthmus overlies the second to the fourth rings of the trachea. Approximately 75% of thyroglossal cysts present as midline swellings. Most fistulae arise after rupture or incision of an infected thyroglossal cyst.

20. C: It receives the two hepatic veins

The IVC is formed by the union of the right and left common iliac veins, behind the right common iliac artery, at the level of L5. It runs to the right of the aorta. It receives the right suprarenal vein directly, but the left suprarenal vein drains into the left renal vein. It opens directly into the right atrium.

21. D: Horner's syndrome

Damage to the T1 root results in a Klumpke's paralysis and is usually caused by a birth injury following traction with the arm extended. The features of this are paralysis of the small muscles of the hand (claw hand), Horner's syndrome (due to traction on the sympathetic chain) and loss of sensation over the medial border of the forearm and hand and over the medial two fingers. An Erb–Duchenne palsy results from damage to the C5 and C6 roots. Wrist drop is caused by damage to the radial nerve (C7/C8) and elbow flexion is mediated by the musculocutaneous nerve (C5/C6).

22. A: Tibialis posterior

Inversion of the foot is effected by the tibialis anterior and tibialis posterior muscles. Flexor hallucis longus assists plantar flexion. Extensor digitorum longus and peroneus longus assist in eversion. Contraction of gastrocnemius causes plantar flexion.

23. **E: Right optic tract**

Lesions at the optic chiasm result in a bitemporal hemianopia. A lesion in the optic radiation causes a contralateral superior homonymous quadrantanopia. A lesion in the optic nerve causes blindness of that eye. Lesions of the optic tract cause a contralateral homonymous hemianopia.

24. **C: Right homonymous hemianopia – left middle cerebral artery occlusion**

Occlusion of the anterior cerebral artery may cause weakness and numbness in the contralateral leg and similar, though milder, symptoms in the arm; the face is spared. Bilateral anterior cerebral artery occlusion is associated with an akinetic mute state due to damage to the cingulate gyri. A homonymous hemianopia can occur as a result of damage to the posterior cerebral artery or to the middle cerebral artery. Contralateral neglect is usually caused by occlusion of the middle cerebral artery of the non-dominant hemisphere. Lateral medullary syndrome is caused by damage to either a vertebral artery or to the posterior inferior cerebellar arteries.

25. **C: Spasticity of muscles on the left side**

The following are features of an upper motor neurone lesion: weakness, spasticity, increased (brisk) tendon reflexes, absent abdominal reflexes and an extensor (up-going) plantar response. In a left-sided cervical spinal cord lesion there will be weakness of the arms and legs and an up-going plantar on that side. Fasciculation of muscles is a lower motor neurone sign.

26. **B: It decussates before leaving the brainstem**

The trochlear nerve supplies the superior oblique muscle. It decussates before leaving the brainstem and runs along the lateral wall of the cavernous sinus. The commonest cause of a lesion in the trochlear nerve is diabetes mellitus and such a lesion would cause slight external rotation of the eyeball.

27. D: Permanent loss of voluntary control of the limb muscles

Complete transection of the cord is usually due to tumour causing cord ischaemia and infarction. There is complete loss of all sensory modalities and paralysis of all voluntary functions below the level of the lesion. This damage is permanent. Reflex activity is regained within six weeks of injury, and it becomes exaggerated.

28. B: Compression of C7 secondary to disc herniation

Nerve roots	Supply
C4/C5	Elbow sensation Supraspinatus
C5/C6	Thumb sensation Biceps
C6/C7	Middle finger sensation Latissumus dorsi Triceps reflex Forearm extensors Wrist extensors/flexors
C7/C8/T1	Little finger sensation Flexor carpi ulnaris Abductor pollicis brevis Interossei Finger extensors

Radial neuropathy at the spiral groove causes sensory loss over the dorsum of the hand but triceps strength is conserved. Ulnar neuropathy at the elbow causes sensory loss in the fourth and fifth digits, as well as weakness of the interossei.

29. D: Constipation

Atropine is an anticholinergic, acting as an antagonist at muscarinic acetylcholine receptors. It causes pupillary dilatation, mild sedation at low doses, agitation and seizures at high doses, reduced gut motility and secretions, tachycardia, bronchodilatation, urinary retention due to bladder wall relaxation, reduced lacrimation and antiparkinsonian effects.

30. E: Dobutamine

The patient is in cardiogenic shock. Noradrenaline acts mainly on α_1 receptors to cause potent vasoconstriction and an increase in systemic vascular resistance. Adrenaline has activity at the β_1 receptor and moderate activity at β_2 and α_1 receptors and is used mainly in anaphylactic shock and as second-line therapy in septic shock. Low-dose dopamine is thought to produce selective renal vasodilatation. Dobutamine is predominantly a β_1 agonist and is used as first-line therapy in cardiogenic shock to increase cardiac output. Phenylephrine is a pure α agonist.

31. B: Mamillary bodies

The limbic system is a collection of connected structures which includes the amygdala, mamillary bodies, hippocampus and certain areas of the cerebrum, such as the cingulated gyrus. Its exact function is unclear but it appears to have a role in the regulation of memory and emotion. Mamillary body atrophy is a relatively specific abnormality found in individuals with a history of Wernicke's encephalopathy and Korsakoff's amnesic syndrome.

32. B: Left-sided lateral medullary syndrome

The lateral medullary syndrome is caused by occlusion of the vertebral artery or of the posterior inferior cerebellar artery, resulting in: vertigo, vomiting, nystagmus towards the side of the lesion, ipsilateral hypotonia, ataxia and paralysis of the soft palate, ipsilateral Horner's syndrome, and loss of pinprick and temperature sensation on the ipsilateral face and contralateral trunk and limbs. The Brown–Séquard syndrome causes ipsilateral loss of proprioception and vibration sensation and contralateral loss of pinprick and temperature sensation. Thalamic infarcts usually involve all sensory modalities. Occlusion of the middle cerebral artery would usually result in motor deficits as well.

Chapter 6
PHYSIOLOGY
Questions

1. A 24-year old woman is admitted to the Accident and Emergency Department with a two-hour history of palpitations. Her electrocardiogram (ECG) reveals a supraventricular tachycardia (SVT). She denies any chest pain, her chest is clear on auscultation, and her blood pressure is 130/76 mmHg. The medical senior house officer on call asks her to perform a Valsalva manoeuvre while some adenosine is being drawn up. Which one of the following physiological responses will occur initially?

- [ ] A A fall in jugular venous pressure
- [ ] B Bradycardia
- [ ] C Increased stroke volume
- [ ] D A fall in systemic blood pressure
- [ ] E A fall in intrathoracic pressure

2. You are phoned by the on-call medical house officer, who has just performed an arterial blood gas on a patient admitted via the Accident and Emergency Department. He is concerned about the following: pH 7.51, Po_2 11.5 kPa, Pco_2 5.3 kPa, serum bicarbonate (HCO_3^-) 38 mmol/l. Which one of the following would be the probable cause?

- [ ] A Treatment with metolazone
- [ ] B Treatment with antiretroviral drugs
- [ ] C Septic shock
- [ ] D Ureterosigmoidostomy
- [ ] E Fanconi syndrome

Answers on page 139

3. You are called to a ward to see a patient who is known to suffer
    from atrial fibrillation. Over the last few hours, the patient has
    become increasingly drowsy, tachycardic and hypotensive. You
    perform a blood gas analysis, which shows a pH of 7.26 and a
    base excess of –10.5 mmol/l. Which one of the following is true
    regarding this picture?

    ☐ A It cannot be present if the arterial pH is normal
    ☐ B The major compensatory mechanism is an increased
          production of HCO_3^- by renal tubular cells
    ☐ C The normal initial response is excretion of CO_2
    ☐ D It is associated with hypokalaemia in all renal tubular acidoses
    ☐ E It is expressed by a rise in the standard HCO_3^- level

4. You are called to see a patient on the ward. He is 43 years old and
    is known to have chronic liver disease. Over the last 30 minutes
    he has vomited about 1.5 litres of bright-red blood. He is
    tachycardic and hypotensive. Acute blood loss of 1.5 litres leads
    to a decrease in which one of the following?

    ☐ A The platelet count
    ☐ B The rate of oxygen extraction by peripheral tissues
    ☐ C The firing rate of carotid and aortic baroreceptors
    ☐ D The cardiac output
    ☐ E Renin secretion

5. A 72-year-old woman comes to the clinic with increasing swelling
    of her legs and exertional breathlessness. She is known to have
    severe ischaemic heart disease. On examination, she has bibasal
    crepitations, a raised jugular venous pulse and bilateral pitting
    oedema up to her waist. An echocardiogram shows a left
    ventricular ejection fraction of 25% and a dilated right heart.
    Which one of the following is a consequence of this clinical
    picture?

    ☐ A Increased sympathetic outflow to the failing heart
    ☐ B Decreased activity of the renin-angiotensin-aldosterone system
    ☐ C Decreased venous pressure
    ☐ D Shift of salt and water from the interstitial space
    ☐ E Widespread vasodilatation

6. A 30-year-old woman has had Crohn's disease for ten years. The disease has run a turbulent course and she has required two laparotomies, the first of which was a hemicolectomy. On the second occasion, a terminal ileal resection for ileocaecal disease was performed. She complains of lethargy at the follow-up clinic. Which one of the following complications is likely to have occurred?

    ☐ A Decreased incidence of gallstone formation
    ☐ B Radiculopathy
    ☐ C Constipation
    ☐ D Pancytopenia
    ☐ E Wernicke's encephalopathy

7. Which one of the following is true regarding the control of ventilation?

    ☐ A Hypoxia reduces the firing of the carotid bodies
    ☐ B Hypercapnia is the main stimulus for breathing in patients with chronic obstructive pulmonary disease (COPD)
    ☐ C Increased arterial Pco_2 increases ventilation mainly by stimulating the central chemoreceptors
    ☐ D The inspiratory neurones are located in the midbrain
    ☐ E Hypoxia stimulates the central chemoreceptors via a rise in $[H^+]$ in the CSF

8. Which one of the following statements about the investigation of respiratory disease is true?

    ☐ A ^{133}Xenon can be used to perform a perfusion scan
    ☐ B Gas transfer factor is usually reduced in pulmonary haemorrhage
    ☐ C Gas transfer factor is usually increased in severe emphysema
    ☐ D Perfusion scanning involves embolisation of the pulmonary vasculature
    ☐ E Gas transfer factor measures the thickness of the alveolar membrane

9. **Which one of the following is true of cortisol?**

☐ A Synthesis occurs in the adrenals via cyclic AMP
☐ B It lacks mineralocorticoid activity
☐ C It inhibits production of angiotensinogen
☐ D It decreases gluconeogenesis
☐ E Plasma levels peak at around midnight

10. **A 68-year-old woman is diagnosed with left ventricular failure and commenced on an ACE inhibitor. Shortly after her first dose of this, she becomes breathless. She deteriorates quickly, developing stridor and facial oedema. As she nears respiratory arrest, urgent anaesthetic help is sought to secure her airway. Which one of the following is an initial consequence of her acute upper airway obstruction?**

☐ A Bradycardia
☐ B Hypercapnia
☐ C A rise in blood pH
☐ D Hypotension
☐ E Wheeze

11. **You are called urgently to a ward. A patient who is receiving a blood transfusion seems to have been given a unit of red cells that had been cross-matched for another patient. The recipient is currently pyrexial, sweaty, breathless and itchy. Which one of the following is true of the ABO and rhesus (Rh) blood grouping systems?**

☐ A If the patient's blood group is AB, his serum will have the naturally occurring anti-A and anti-B antibodies
☐ B Naturally occurring anti-A and anti-B antibodies are usually IgG
☐ C Fewer than 10% of Caucasians are Rh-positive
☐ D The presence of the D antigen makes the subject Rh-positive
☐ E Rhesus antibodies are naturally occurring antibodies

12. A 49-year-old man with known diabetic nephropathy attends his six-monthly appointment at the Renal Outpatients Clinic. His baseline creatinine is 340 μmol/l, which is unchanged on this visit. He complains of increased lethargy, and blood tests reveal a haemoglobin of 7.4 g/dl. His mean corpuscular volume (MCV) and haematinics are within normal limits and, because he has already had several iron infusions, you discuss the idea of commencing erythropoeitin injections. Which one of the following statements is true of erythropoiesis and erythropoietin?

☐ A Hypoxia is the main stimulus to erythropoietin production
☐ B Erythropoietin increases the maturation time for red cell precursors
☐ C Erythropoietin levels are found to be low in secondary polycythaemia
☐ D Bilateral nephrectomy completely abolishes erythropoietin production
☐ E Erythropoietin is produced by δ-aminolaevulinic acid synthetase (ALA-S)

13. Which one of the following statements about the control of the peripheral circulation and blood pressure is true?

☐ A Carotid chemoreceptors have no role in the control of blood pressure
☐ B The sudden assumption of an upright posture increases venous return
☐ C The sudden assumption of an upright posture results in a bradycardia
☐ D The central vasomotor centre is situated in the medulla oblongata
☐ E The arterioles account for about 90% of total peripheral resistance

14. Which one of the following statements about vasoactive intestinal peptide (VIP) is true?

☐ A It stimulates gastric acid secretion
☐ B Its normal serum level is 3000 ng/l
☐ C It may be secreted by a bronchogenic carcinoma
☐ D It enhances small intestinal reabsorption of water and electrolytes
☐ E It is secreted by β islet cells in the pancreas

15. A 40-year-old man attends the Liver Clinic. He has chronic liver disease caused by chronic alcohol abuse and was recently admitted with an episode of acute decompensation. At that time his prothrombin time was prolonged and he was started on vitamin K supplements, intravenously at first, and now by mouth. He asks you if he can now stop taking this. Which one of the following statements about vitamin K is true?

☐ A The commonest cause of vitamin K deficiency is dietary lack
☐ B Oral supplements cannot be absorbed in the absence of bile salts
☐ C It is a biological antioxidant
☐ D Warfarin inhibits the vitamin-K dependent carboxylation of factors I, V and XI in the liver
☐ E Vitamin K reverses the effects of warfarin instantaneously

16. Which one of the following is true regarding the physiological mechanisms which occur after trauma to a blood vessel?

☐ A Minute ruptures in small vessels are always sealed by blood clots
☐ B Platelet aggregation can be inhibited by ADP and thrombin
☐ C The temporary platelet plug is converted to a blood clot by thrombin
☐ D The endothelium produces prostacyclin to stimulate platelet adhesion
☐ E The endothelium produces thromboxane A_2 to inhibit platelet adhesion

17. A 35-year-old woman has Raynaud's disease. It is so severe that she cannot expose her hands to any cool temperatures without suffering excruciating pain. A successful sympathectomy is carried out to the hand. Which one of the following effects will occur as a result of this procedure?

☐ A There is a permanent abolition of sweating
☐ B There is a permanent increase in blood flow
☐ C Existing ischaemia will not improve
☐ D The skin responds only to central temperature changes
☐ E The skin does not respond to local temperature changes

18. Which one of the following inhibits the secretion of antidiuretic hormone (ADH)?

☐ A Alcohol
☐ B Nicotine
☐ C Pain
☐ D Exercise
☐ E Emotional stress

19. Which one of the following statements about bilirubin and its metabolites is true?

☐ A In a 70-kg adult the daily production of bilirubin is about 3 mg
☐ B A fraction of urobilinogen is reabsorbed from the intestine and re-excreted through the liver
☐ C Urobilinogen is orange in colour
☐ D Conjugated bilirubin enters the bile by simple diffusion
☐ E The conjugation of bilirubin is catalysed by the enzyme β-glucuronidase

Answers on pages 143–144   123

20. Which one of the following statements about potassium homeostasis is true?

- [ ] A Hypokalaemia directly stimulates aldosterone secretion
- [ ] B Insulin causes potassium loss from the cells
- [ ] C 20% of total body potassium is located in the extracellular space
- [ ] D If the membrane-bound ATP-dependent sodium pump is impaired, hypokalaemia will result
- [ ] E Aldosterone increases active potassium secretion in the distal convoluted tubule

21. Which one of the following statements about carbon dioxide (CO_2) in the blood is most true?

- [ ] A Pco_2 is usually higher than normal in compensated metabolic acidosis
- [ ] B Pco_2 is usually lower than normal in compensated metabolic alkalosis
- [ ] C For a given pH, the Pco_2 is inversely proportional to $[HCO_3^-]$
- [ ] D Most of the CO_2 in blood is present in the form of H_2CO_3
- [ ] E The main buffer for H^+ generated by the entry of CO_2 into red blood cells is haemoglobin

22. Which one of the following statements about hydrogen ion (H^+) homeostasis is true?

- [ ] A Phosphates are the most important buffers in the extracellular fluid
- [ ] B Proteins are the main buffer in urine
- [ ] C Ammonium ions (NH_4^+) cannot cross the renal tubular cell membrane
- [ ] D The H^+ ion concentration ($[H^+]$) is inversely proportional to the Pco_2
- [ ] E H^+ ions are secreted into the renal tubular lumen in exchange for K^+ ions, and combine with the filtered bicarbonate

23. A 28-year-old woman is admitted with suspected meningoencephalitis and commenced on intravenous ceftriaxone and aciclovir. She deteriorates rapidly and is admitted to the Intensive Care Unit with multi-organ failure. Her urine output drops steadily and her serum creatinine rises to 687 μmol/l. Which one of the following should be kept in mind when prescribing her antimicrobial drugs?

☐ A Her true glomerular filtration rate (GFR) will be higher than her creatinine clearance

☐ B The Cockcroft–Gault formula will underestimate her GFR if she is obese

☐ C The serum urea is a more accurate index of GFR than the serum creatinine

☐ D Her creatinine clearance should not be used as a guide

☐ E The creatinine clearance is inversely proportional to the serum creatinine concentration

24. Which one of the following is true of the healthy nephron?

☐ A ADH renders the cells lining the proximal tubule permeable to water

☐ B All filtered glucose is reabsorbed in the proximal tubule

☐ C Most filtered protein is reabsorbed in the distal convoluted tubule

☐ D The descending loop of Henle is impermeable to water

☐ E 20% of filtered sodium is reabsorbed by the nephron

25. Which one of the following provides a good assessment of GFR?

☐ A Serum β_2-microglobulin
☐ B Serum albumin
☐ C Serum urea
☐ D Amino acid chromatography of urine
☐ E Water deprivation test

26. A 23-year-old man with type 1 diabetes is brought in to Casualty fitting. He has been unwell with diarrhoea and vomiting for a few days and has been off his food, but he has continued to take his insulin. His glucose level on admission is 0.9 mmol/l. Which one of the following is most true regarding his current physiological state?

- [ ] A There will be decreased cortisol secretion
- [ ] B Growth hormone secretion will be inhibited
- [ ] C TSH secretion will be decreased
- [ ] D There will be decreased adrenaline (epinephrine) secretion
- [ ] E Glucagon secretion will be increased

27. Which one of the following shifts the oxygen dissociation curve to the left?

- [ ] A Sickle cell anaemia
- [ ] B Decreased intracellular concentration of 2,3-diphosphoglycerate (2,3-DPG)
- [ ] C Pyrexia
- [ ] D Hypercapnia
- [ ] E Metabolic acidosis

28. Which one of the following happens when the renin–angiotensin system is stimulated by hypovolaemic shock?

- [ ] A Angiotensin-converting enzymes degrade bradykinin
- [ ] B Angiotensin II stimulates the adrenal cortex to increase cortisol production
- [ ] C Renin converts angiotensin I into angiotensin II
- [ ] D Angiotensin I stimulates the adrenal medulla to synthesise aldosterone
- [ ] E Angiotensin II causes vasoconstriction of the efferent glomerular arteriole

29. Which one of the following effects is caused by insulin?

- [ ] A Decreased glucose uptake by muscle
- [ ] B Increased protein synthesis
- [ ] C Decreased glycogen synthesis
- [ ] D Increased ketogenesis in the liver
- [ ] E Increased lipolysis in adipose tissue

30. Which one of the following statements about hormones and pregnancy is most true?

- [ ] A β-Human chorionic gonadotrophin (HCG) is detectable in blood four weeks after conception
- [ ] B A low serum progesterone in pregnancy is associated with recurrent abortion
- [ ] C Cortisol and corticosterone are produced by the placenta in the second trimester
- [ ] D HCG becomes undetectable in urine in the third trimester
- [ ] E The function of the corpus luteum is vital until the third trimester

31. Which one of the following factors stimulates renin release?

- [ ] A Propranolol
- [ ] B Angiotensin II
- [ ] C Salt depletion
- [ ] D An increase in blood pressure
- [ ] E An increase in plasma potassium concentration

32. Which of the following is true regarding the blood–brain barrier?

- [ ] A Water-soluble compounds tend to cross it more quickly
- [ ] B Proteins and glucose cross readily
- [ ] C It allows transport from the blood to the brain only
- [ ] D It lacks mitochondria in the endothelial cells
- [ ] E It is poorly developed at birth

Answers on pages 146–148

33. A 35-year-old woman presents to the Accident and Emergency Department with a two-month history of severe occipital headaches with associated photophobia and vomiting. There is a family history of migraines. She undergoes a CT scan of her brain and a lumbar puncture, which fail to reveal any abnormality. Which one of the following is likely to be present in her cerebrospinal fluid (CSF)?

A Glucose at a level less than one third of that in blood
B About 10 polymorphs/mm³
C Immunoglobulin
D Oligoclonal bands
E 0.02–0.04 g/l of protein

34. Which one of the following is true of the electromyogram (EMG)?

A It shows fibrillation potentials in denervated muscle
B It is usually recorded by placing electrodes within the muscle fibres
C It requires a general anaesthetic to be administered
D It records the magnitude of muscle contraction
E It shows regular electrical activity when healthy muscle is relaxed

35. Which one of the following factors decreases cerebral blood flow?

A Seizures
B Inhalation of hyperbaric oxygen
C Inhalation of 7% CO_2
D Chronic anaemia
E Intraventricular administration of noradrenaline (norepinephrine)

36. **Which one of the following sensory modalities is transmitted by the spinothalamic tracts of the spinal cord?**

- [ ] A Temperature
- [ ] B Joint position
- [ ] C Vibration
- [ ] D Two-point discrimination
- [ ] E Proprioception

37. **Which one of the following autonomic neurones are adrenergic?**

- [ ] A Post-ganglionic parasympathetic neurones to the stomach
- [ ] B Post-ganglionic sympathetic neurones to the small bowel
- [ ] C Autonomic pre-ganglionic neurones
- [ ] D Post-ganglionic sympathetic neurones to the sweat glands
- [ ] E The parasympathetic fibres supplying the sphincter pupillae of the iris

38. **Which one of the following is under parasympathetic control in the autonomic nervous system?**

- [ ] A Ejaculation
- [ ] B Gallbladder relaxation
- [ ] C An increase in atrial contractility
- [ ] D Detrusor muscle relaxation
- [ ] E Ciliary muscle contraction

39. **Which one of the following inhibits the secretion of gastrin?**

- [ ] A Hypercalcaemia
- [ ] B A protein meal
- [ ] C Gastric distension
- [ ] D Increased gastric acidity
- [ ] E Increased vagal activity

Answers on pages 149–150   129

40. Which one of the following statements about the electrocardiogram (ECG) is true?

☐ A The opening of the aortic valve coincides with the P wave
☐ B Isovolumetric contraction occurs during the P wave
☐ C During the T wave the tricuspid valve is normally open
☐ D During the ST segment all parts of the ventricle have been depolarised
☐ E The QT interval may be prolonged in hyperkalaemia

41. A 39-year-old man presents with a one-month history of worsening headaches, visual disturbances and nausea. He is intubated and ventilated because of a deterioration in his level of conciousness and he undergoes a CT brain scan. This is reported as: 'There is a 2 cm × 2 cm mass in the right parietal lobe. There is effacement of the ventricles and loss of the sulci. Appearances are suggestive of a primary astrocytoma with raised intracranial pressure.' Which one of the following could be used to decrease the intracranial pressure in the first instance?

☐ A Administration of labetolol
☐ B Administration of propofol
☐ C Intravenous diazepam
☐ D Hyperventilation
☐ E Nursing the patient in the head-down position

42. Which one of the following substances decreases intestinal secretion of water and electrolytes?

☐ A Noradrenaline (norepinephrine)
☐ B Vasoactive intestinal polypeptide (VIP)
☐ C Prostaglandins
☐ D Dihydroxy bile acids
☐ E Acetylcholine

43. **Which one of the following statements about the digestion and absorption of fat is true?**

    ☐ A A low pH enhances pancreatic lipase action
    ☐ B Long-chain triglycerides are more water-soluble than medium-chain triglycerides
    ☐ C Bile salts act as emulsifying agents
    ☐ D Cholesterol from micelles enters mucosal cells by active transport
    ☐ E On a moderate fat intake, over 50% of ingested fat is absorbed

44. **Which one of the following is true of pain?**

    ☐ A It is transmitted through the posterior columns of the spinal cord
    ☐ B Visceral pain is always well localised
    ☐ C If intractable, it may be relieved by lobotomy
    ☐ D It is transmitted faster through C fibres than through A fibres
    ☐ E Transmission is facilitated by the stimulation of μ (mu) receptors in the CNS

45. **Which one of the following is true of luteinising hormone releasing-hormone (LHRH)?**

    ☐ A It exerts negative feedback on follicle-stimulating hormone (FSH) and on luteinising hormone (LH)
    ☐ B It is used in the treatment of infertility in women only
    ☐ C It produces a greater response in LH release when given intravenously during the early follicular phase than when it is given during the luteal phase
    ☐ D It is secreted by the pituitary in a pulsatile fashion
    ☐ E Its analogues may be used in the treatment of prostatic carcinoma

Answers on pages 150–153

46. **Which one of the following statements about the mechanism of vomiting is correct?**

- [ ] A The chemoreceptor trigger zone (CTZ) is protected by the blood–brain barrier
- [ ] B Anticholinergic drugs inhibit vomiting by acting mainly on the CTZ
- [ ] C Stimulation of H_1 receptors in the vestibular system inhibits vomiting
- [ ] D The main receptors in the CTZ are dopaminergic (D_2)
- [ ] E 5-hydroxytryptamine (5-HT_3) agonists are effective in the control of cis-platinum-induced vomiting

47. **Which one of the following is true of adult haemoglobin?**

- [ ] A It contains four globin molecules
- [ ] B It binds carbon dioxide (CO_2) irreversibly to form carboxyhaemoglobin
- [ ] C It has a higher affinity for carbon monoxide (CO) than for oxygen
- [ ] D It carries ionic rather than molecular oxygen
- [ ] E Its production is decreased indirectly by hypoxia

48. **Which one of the following is true of the QRS complex of the electrocardiogram?**

- [ ] A It may be used to assess the rotation of the heart along its longitudinal axis
- [ ] B It is shortened in tricyclic antidepressant poisoning
- [ ] C It is caused by ventricular myocardial repolarisiation
- [ ] D It will normally contain a Q wave up to half the height of the R wave
- [ ] E It corresponds to atrial systole

49. A 53-year-old woman is referred by her general practitioner. She had a bout of diarrhoea and vomiting one month ago. Now she is complaining of increasing weakness of her arms and legs. On examination, she has marked weakness of her arms and legs and bilateral ptosis. She also appears to be breathing in a shallow pattern. It is suspected that she has Guillain–Barré syndrome with respiratory muscle involvement. Which one of the following is true of her pattern of respiratory muscle weakness?

- A   The ratio of forced expiratory volume in one second (FEV_1) to vital capacity (VC) is reduced
- B   The ratio of residual volume (RV) to total lung capacity (TLC) is decreased
- C   Gas transfer (corrected for lung volume) is reduced
- D   Hypercapnia is an early feature
- E   The VC falls when the patient is moved from an upright to a supine position

50. Which one of the following causes vasodilatation of the peripheral arterial blood vessels?

- A   Endothelin
- B   Prostaglandins
- C   Angiotensin
- D   Thromboxane A_2
- E   Adenosine diphosphate

51. Which one of the following is true of leptin?

- A   Its actions generally cause weight gain
- B   Its levels are low in obese individuals
- C   It is secreted by the hypothalamus
- D   It suppresses appetite
- E   It is a product of the MHC gene

52. **Consider the following diagram representing subdivisions of the lung volume:**

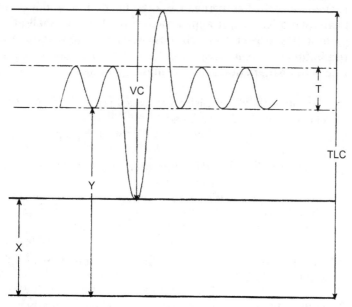

T = resting tidal volume; VC = vital capacity; TLC = total lung capacity; X and Y represent volumes

Which one of the following statements is true with regards to this diagram?

- A X is the functional residual capacity
- B Y is the expiratory reserve volume
- C TLC can be measured using a simple spirometer
- D A general anaesthetic increases Y
- E X is increased in a patient with emphysema

53. **A 22-year-old medical student is part of an expedition group trekking in Northern India. The group fly to the mountain plateau of Ladakh, which is approximately 14,000 feet in altitude, to start their ascent. Over the next 24 hours, he begins to develop a headache, nausea and vomiting. The team medic examines his chest and thinks that she can hear bibasal crepitations. Which one of the following statements about his body's physiological response to the atmospheric conditions at altitude is true?**

- [ ] A   He is likely to have a respiratory acidosis
- [ ] B   The cerebral blood flow will decrease due to vasocontriction
- [ ] C   There will be increased atrial naturetic peptide release
- [ ] D   There will be a marked reduction in ventilation
- [ ] E   The pulmonary artery pressure falls dramatically

54. **A 23-year old professional footballer attends the Cardiology Outpatients Clinic, having been referred by his general practitioner with a six-month history of exertional breathlessness and atypical chest pain. He feels that his exercise tolerance and performance on the field have deteriorated considerably of late. During his last game, he had an episode of dizziness and lost consciousness for a matter of seconds. An echocardiogram is performed, which reveals significant hypertrophy of the interventricular septum, systolic anterior motion of the mitral valve (SAM) and a left ventricular outflow tract gradient of 40 mmHg at rest. Which one of the following is true of the abnormality which has been dicovered?**

- [ ] A   Amyl nitrite will result in a reduced left ventricular (LV) outflow tract obstruction
- [ ] B   A reduction in afterload will improve the outflow tract obstruction
- [ ] C   A reduction in pre-load will improve the outflow tract obstruction
- [ ] D   LV outflow tract obstruction will be increased by leg elevation
- [ ] E   Fever and exercise will both reduce the outflow tract obstruction

55. A 71-year-old man with known mild congestive cardiac failure is admitted with acute shortness of breath and chest pain. He is usually on 20 mg of furosemide (frusemide) a day. His general practitioner has also recently diagnosed gout and commenced him on diclofenac as required. On arrival he is distressed, and examination reveals widespread bilateral coarse crepitations in the chest. An ECG shows new T-wave inversion throughout the precordial leads. An arterial blood gas shows the following results: pH 7.12, Po_2 5.6 kPa, Pco_2 6.78 kPa; plasma lactate 5.7 mmol/l. Which one of the following statements is most likely to be true?

- [ ] A Intravenous diuretic is the best treatment for improving cardiac output
- [ ] B Intravenous nitrates would lead to a reduction in stroke volume
- [ ] C The diclofenac has probably caused a drop in cardiac contractility
- [ ] D Furosemide will increase the left ventricular end-diastolic pressure
- [ ] E There is additional pathology present which is causing a lactic acidosis

56. A 21-year-old man is admitted via the Accident and Emergency Department with a history of lethargy, malaise and haemoptysis. Blood tests reveal the following: haemoglobin 7.5 g/dl, Na^+ 136 mmol/l, K^+ 7.8 mmol/l, urea 23.5 mmol/l, creatinine 456 μmol/l. A chest X-ray shows bilateral basal air-space shadowing and urine microscopy reveals the presence of protein and red cell casts. Which one of the following is most likely to be present?

- [ ] A An increased diffusion capacity of carbon monoxide (TLCO)
- [ ] B A significant lung perfusion defect
- [ ] C A reduced peak expiratory flow rate
- [ ] D A respiratory acidosis
- [ ] E A metabolic alkalosis

57. A 39-year-old woman presents to her general practitioner with a history of tiredness. He performs a thorough physical examination and fails to detect any abnormal findings. A full blood screen is performed, including a complete endocrine profile. The results of these tests show several abnormalities: TSH 20.5 mU/l, free thyroxine (FT4) 1.1 pmol/l, prolactin 1020 U/l. Which of the following is the most likely diagnosis?

- [ ] A Pituitary adenoma
- [ ] B Hypothyroidism
- [ ] C Sick euthyroid syndrome
- [ ] D Subclinical hypothyroidism
- [ ] E Pregnancy

PHYSIOLOGY

Answers

1. **D: A fall in systemic blood pressure**

    The Valsalva manoeuvre is forced expiration against a closed glottis. It causes an increase in intrapulmonary and intrathoracic pressure and thus impedes venous return to the heart. This causes a transient decrease in stroke volume and blood pressure. On release, there is a sudden increase in venous return, an increase in blood pressure and a slowing of the heart rate.

2. **A: Treatment with metolazone**

    The actual bicarbonate level ([HCO_3^-]) is 23–33 mmol/l. An elevated plasma HCO_3^- concentration can result from metabolic alkalosis or from the secondary metabolic response to respiratory acidosis. The projectile vomiting of pyloric stenosis results in hydrogen ion (H^+) loss and metabolic alkalosis. Other causes of a metabolic alkalosis include excess oral intake of alkali or forced alkaline diuresis and thiazide or loop diuretic therapy. Metabolic acidosis (low serum [HCO_3^-]) is a feature of diabetic ketoacidosis, ureterosigmoidostomy and renal tubular acidosis. Drugs such as metformin and antiretrovirals can cause a lactic acidosis, as can any form of shock secondary to organ hypoperfusion.

3. **C: The normal initial response is excretion of CO_2**

    The normal initial response to a metabolic acidosis is an increased respiratory rate in an attempt to excrete CO_2:

$$H^+ + HCO_3^- \leftrightarrow H_2CO_3 \rightarrow H_2O + CO_2$$

This respiratory compensation reduces serum bicarbonate and elevates pH. The renal compensatory mechanisms then bring about the excretion of extra H^+ to bring the buffer system back to equilibrium. Hyperkalaemia is a feature of type 4 renal tubular acidosis.

4. **C: The firing rate of carotid and aortic baroreceptors**

Acute hypovolaemia causes hypotension. This causes inhibition of baroreceptors, which in turn causes a rise in systemic vascular resistance. Hypotension also stimulates secretion of renin, which increases the availability of angiotensins (vasopressors) and aldosterone (salt and water retention). The rate of oxygen extraction, the cardiac output and the platelet count would all rise.

5. **A: Increased sympathetic outflow to the failing heart**

The reduced cardiac output stimulates the sympathetic system via the baroreceptors. The decreased renal perfusion stimulates the renin-angiotensin-aldosterone system, which increases vasoconstriction. The Starling curve moves downwards when the heart fails.

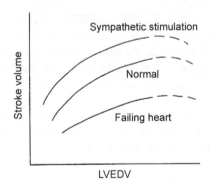

6. **D: Pancytopenia**

    The function of the terminal ileum is the absorption of vitamin B_{12} and bile salts. Deficiency of vitamin B_{12} may result in pancytopenia, peripheral neuropathy and subacute combined degeneration of the cord. Bile salt malabsorption increases the incidence of gallstones and reduces fat digestion and absorption. Diarrhoea results from fatty stools and colonic irritation by bile salts.

7. **C: Increased arterial Pco_2 increases ventilation mainly by stimulating the central chemoreceptors**

    The central regulatory centres that control the rate and depth of respiration are located in the medulla and pons. The carotid body chemoreceptors respond to a decrease in arterial Po_2, a high Pco_2 and a low pH. The aortic body chemoreceptors respond to increased Pco_2 and low Po_2. Carbon dioxide stimulates the central chemoreceptors by an increase of Pco_2 ([H+]) in the CSF. Hypoxia is the main stimulus to the respiratory drive in patients with chronic obstructive pulmonary disease.

8. **D: Perfusion scanning involves embolisation of the pulmonary vasculature**

    The ventilation part of a ventilation-perfusion scan involves the inhalation of one of several available radio-labelled gases, such as ^{133}Xe. The perfusion part involves the injection of radio-labelled albumin microspheres which embolise in the pulmonary microvasculature. Measurement of gas transfer factor determines how efficiently oxygen is transferred from the alveolus to the red cell, and depends on thickness of the alveolar membrane. The gas transfer factor is reduced in infiltrative lung disease, pulmonary fibrosis, multiple pulmonary emboli and emphysema. It may be increased in asthmatics, hyperkinetic states, pulmonary haemorrhage, polycythaemia and in left-to-right shunts.

9.   A: Synthesis occurs in the adrenals via cyclic AMP

ACTH blinds to special receptors on the plasma membrane of
adrenocortical cells, causing an increase in intracellular cAMP and
activation of protein kinase A. Cortisol has a circadian rhythm and
levels are highest in the morning (around 08.00 am) and lowest
around midnight. Cortisol has several anti-insulin actions,
including stimulation of glycogenesis and gluconeogenesis from
protein (both in the liver). It also increases protein catabolism,
lipolysis and free fatty acid mobilisation, and has some
mineralocorticoid activity.

10.   B: Hypercapnia

In acute airway obstruction, the classic signs of cyanosis and
inspiratory stridor are found. Hypoxia and hypercapnia occur
simultaneously. Initially, there is tachycardia and hypertension as a
result of the stress response but hypotension and bradycardia
develop later on.

11.   D: The presence of the D antigen makes the subject Rh-positive

A subject whose blood group is AB does not have anti-A and anti-B
antibodies. The naturally occurring antibodies are usually IgM.
Around 80% of Caucasians are Rh-positive, while Japanese and
Africans are usually Rh-negative. Rh antibodies are immune
antibodies.

12.   A: Hypoxia is the main stimulus to erythropoietin production

Hypoxia is the chief stimulus to erythropoiesis. Around 85% of
erythropoietin (166 amino acids) is produced by the kidneys and
15% is produced by the liver. The rate-controlling enzyme for
porphyrin and haem synthesis is ALA-S. Its synthesis is inhibited by
haemoglobin in polycythaemia rubra vera. Genetically engineered
erythropoietin is now available for the treatment of anaemia
caused by renal failure.

13. D: The central vasomotor centre is situated in the medulla oblongata

Hypoxia stimulates the carotid chemoreceptors, causing tachycardia and vasoconstriction and an elevation in blood pressure. Sudden assumption of the upright posture results in a fall in venous return, stroke volume, cardiac output and blood pressure. This stimulates the sympathetic system, which causes constriction of medium-sized veins and a decrease in the firing rate of the carotid and aortic baroreceptors (stretch receptors). The compensatory response is an increase in heart rate and in peripheral resistance. Arterioles account for about 40% of total peripheral resistance.

14. C: It may be secreted by a bronchogenic carcinoma

VIP (28 amino acids) stimulates the intestinal secretion of water and electrolytes. It inhibits gastric acid secretion and causes peripheral vasodilatation. VIPomas result in the Verner–Morrison or WDHA syndrome (**w**atery **d**iarrhoea, **h**ypokalaemia and **a**chlorhydria).

15. B: Oral supplements cannot be absorbed in the absence of bile salts

Vitamin K is a fat-soluble vitamin and deficiency occurs in fat-malabsorption states. Warfarin inhibits vitamin K-epoxide reductase, thereby inhibiting the formation of the reduced form of vitamin K (KH_2). This reduced form is the cofactor for decarboxylation of glutamate residues in the inactive pro-enzyme forms of factors X, IX, VII and II in the liver. It takes approximately 21 hours for vitamin K to reverse warfarin effects.

16. C: The temporary platelet plug is converted to a blood clot by thrombin

Injury to the wall of a blood vessel causes contraction and platelet aggregation. This temporary haemostatic plug is converted to a definitive plug by thrombin. Minute ruptures in small vessels are often sealed by a platelet plug rather than by a blood clot. The vascular endothelium produces prostacyclin which inhibits platelet adhesion.

17. **A: There is a permanent abolition of sweating**

   The section of the hand's sympathetic nerve supply causes complete abolition of sweating. Skin ischaemia, if present, may improve. Immediately after sympathectomy there is increased blood flow due to vasodilatation, but this increase is not maintained permanently. Sympathectomy renders the skin unresponsive to central temperature changes, but it will still respond to local temperature changes.

18. **A: Alcohol**

   Stimuli to ADH secretion include: increased osmotic pressure of the plasma, emotional stress, surgical trauma, pain, morphine, nicotine and barbiturates. Release of ADH can occur in response to an increase in osmolarity (via stimulation of osmoreceptors located in the anterior hypothalamus) or to a decreased fluid volume (via a decrease in the stretch of the volume receptors located in the left atrium, vena cavae, carotid sinus and aortic arch).

19. **B: A fraction of urobilinogen is reabsorbed from the intestine and re-excreted through the liver**

   Bilirubin is formed from the catabolism of the haem moiety of the haemoglobin molecule, and is transported to the liver bound to albumin. Bilirubin is conjugated with glucuronic acid, catalysed by glucuronyl transferase, to form water-soluble bilirubin diglucuronide, which is excreted into the bile canaliculi via an active process. The conjugated bilirubin is converted by intestinal bacteria into unconjugated bilirubin and urobilinogens (colourless compounds), which are reabsorbed by the intestinal mucosa. Some of the reabsorbed substances are re-excreted by the liver (enterohepatic circulation).

20. E: Aldosterone increases active potassium secretion in the distal convoluted tubule

Hyperkalaemia stimulates aldosterone secretion, which increases potassium secretion into the distal convoluted tubule. Insulin causes potassium to enter the cells. Only around 2% of total body potassium is located in the extracellular space. Impairment of the ATP-dependent sodium pump causes potassium to accumulate extracellularly, resulting in hyperkalaemia.

21. E: The main buffer for H^+ generated by the entry of CO_2 into red blood cells is haemoglobin

The partial pressure of CO_2 is directly proportional to the concentration of HCO_3^- (where k is the dissociation coefficient of carbonic acid):

$$Pco_2 = pH \times k \times [HCO_3^-]$$

In a metabolic alkalosis, the respiratory system attempts to compensate for metabolic alkalosis by retaining CO_2 in order to restore blood pH. Most of the CO_2 in blood is in the form of bicarbonate.

22. C: Ammonium ions (NH_4^+) cannot cross the renal tubular cell membrane

Bicarbonate is the most important buffer in the extracellular fluid, whereas phosphate is the main buffer in urine. Ammonium ions (NH_4^+) cannot cross cell membranes because of their electrical charge, but ammonia (NH_3) can. The pH is related to the [HCO_3^-] as follows (where pK is the dissociation constant of the buffer, 6.10 at body temperature):

$$pH = pK + \log \frac{[HCO_3^-]}{[H_2CO_3]}$$

H^+ is secreted into the renal tubule in exchange for Na^+.

23. **E: The creatinine clearance is inversely proportional to the serum creatinine concentration**

   The creatinine clearance is higher than the true GFR because of active secretion of creatinine in the renal tubules. The Cockcroft–Gault formula tends to overestimate creatinine clearance in obese patients as endogenous creatinine production will be less than predicted by body weight. The level of serum urea is affected by many factors outside the kidney and is therefore a less accurate index of GFR than serum creatnine.

24. **B: All filtered glucose is reabsorbed in the proximal tubule**

   It is the ascending loop of Henle that is impermeable to water. Aldosterone controls Na^+ reabsorption in exchange for H^+ and K^+ in the distal convoluted tubule. Filtered protein is reabsorbed in the proximal convoluted tubule. ADH acts on the collecting ducts to render them permeable to water. Approximately 99% of filtered sodium is reabsorbed.

25. **A: Serum β_2-microglobulin**

   Amino acid chromatography assesses proximal tubule function. The water deprivation test assesses distal tubule function.

26. **E: Glucagon secretion will be increased**

   Hypoglycaemia stimulates the release of glucocorticoids, growth hormone, catecholamines and TSH. Glucagon stimulates glycogenolysis by acting on hepatocytes, causing an increase in intracellular cAMP and cytoplasmic Ca^{2+}.

27. **B: Decreased intracellular concentration of 2,3-diphosphoglycerate (2,3-DPG)**

   The oxygen saturation of haemoglobin is related to the partial pressure of oxygen in arterial blood by the oxygen dissociation curve. When the curve shifts to the right, for a given partial pressure of oxygen there is a decreased affinity of haemoglobin for oxygen. This occurs with increased Pco_2, increased temperature and acidosis (where haemoglobin needs to give up oxygen more readily to metabolically active tissues). The oxygen dissociation curve is pushed to the left by a low concentration of 2,3-DPG. The production of 2,3-DPG is stimulated by hypoxia due to high altitude or to anaemia, which shifts the curve to the right.

28. A: Angiotensin-converting enzymes degrade bradykinin

Renin converts angiotensin into angiotensin I, which is converted to angiotensin II by the converting enzymes. Angiotensin II is vasoactive and stimulates aldosterone secretion and depresses renin output. The use of angiotensin-converting enzyme inhibitors results in bradykinin accumulation, which manifests as a troublesome cough in some individuals.

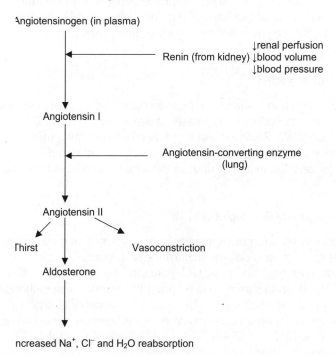

Angiotensinogen (in plasma)

Renin (from kidney) ↓renal perfusion ↓blood volume ↓blood pressure

Angiotensin I

Angiotensin-converting enzyme (lung)

Angiotensin II

Thirst   Vasoconstriction

Aldosterone

Increased Na^+, Cl^- and H_2O reabsorption

147

29. B: Increased protein synthesis

Insulin decreases lipolysis and ketogenesis and increases glycogenesis and glucose uptake by the cells. It also has an anabolic effect on proteins. (See also the answer to Question 8, Clinical Chemistry.)

30. B: A low serum progesterone in pregnancy is associated with recurrent abortion

HCG is detectable in blood as early as six days after conception and can sometimes be measured in the urine as early as 14 days after conception. The urinary levels of HCG begin to fall around the 11th week, but remain detectable throughout the pregnancy. Cortisol is produced in the fetal adrenal glands. The placenta produces enough oestrogen and progesterone to take over the function of the corpus luteum after the sixth week of pregnancy and its function begins to decline after the eighth week.

31. C: Salt depletion

Renin secretion is stimulated by a decrease in the circulating blood volume, catecholamines, potassium depletion and the oral contraceptive. Renin release is reduced by hypernatraemia, hyperkalaemia, angiotensin II, ADH, ACE inhibitors and β-blockers. Renin acts to raise blood pressure and blood volume.

32. E: It is poorly developed at birth

Lipid-soluble substances, oxygen, carbon dioxide and water are able to cross the blood–brain barrier easily. Water-soluble substances, however, cross with difficulty. The endothelial cells of the blood–brain barrier have six times the number of mitochondria of normal endothelial cells. There are bi-directional transport systems and proteins cross to a very limited degree, while glucose crosses slowly. The blood–brain barrier is more permeable at birth and develops during the early years of life. This is demonstrated by the fact that damage to the basal ganglia occurs in jaundiced neonates (kernicterus) but not in adults.

33. **C: Immunoglobulin**

   CSF glucose concentration is normally more than 50% of that of blood. A low CSF glucose is found in bacterial, tuberculous and fungal meningitis. The normal CSF contains mononuclear cells only (around 5/mm^3). Oligoclonal bands are abnormal and may indicate CNS disease, for example multiple sclerosis. The normal CSF protein concentration is 0.15–0.45 g/l. Immunoglobulin is present in healthy CSF.

34. **A: It shows fibrillation potentials in denervated muscle**

   Electromyography (EMG) is usually recorded using small metal discs on the skin overlying the muscle. It is also possible to use hypodermic needle electrodes and pick up the activity in single muscle fibres. There is no recordable electrical activity in relaxed healthy muscle. The EMG does not measure the magnitude of muscle contraction.

35. **B: Inhalation of hyperbaric oxygen**

   The factors which increase cerebral blood flow are seizures, hypoxia, hypercapnia, chronic anaemia and intraventricular noradrenaline (norepinephrine). A local increase in Po_2 or a decrease in Pco_2 have a vasoconstrictor effect on cerebral vessels.

36. **A: Temperature**

   The spinothalamic tracts transmit pain and temperature signals. Joint-position (proprioception), two-point discrimination and vibration sensations are carried by the posterior columns. Fine touch is transmitted by both pathways and so is not a useful discrimination test in the clinical setting.

37. **B: Post-ganglionic sympathetic neurones to the small bowel**

   Post-ganglionic sympathetic neurones to the sweat glands, autonomic pre-ganglionic neurones and parasympathetic fibres to smooth muscle are cholinergic.

38. E: Ciliary muscle contraction

Ejaculation is sympathetically mediated (it is erection which is a parasympathetic function). Parasympathetic function decreases atrial contractility and causes contraction of the detrusor muscle, the gallbladder and ciliary muscle.

See Table opposite

39. D: Increased gastric acidity

Gastrin is secreted from the G cells of the gastric antrum. Its actions are to increase the secretion of gastric acid and pepsin, encourage gastric emptying and increase the secretion of insulin and glucagons from the pancreas. Stimuli for gastrin release include amino acids in the antrum, vagal action and distension of the antrum by food. Gastrin secretion is inhibited by a pH of less than 1.5, gastric acid and secretin.

40. D: During the ST segment all parts of the ventricle have been depolarised

Isovolumetric contraction occurs during ventricular systole when the mitral and tricuspid valves are closed. It lasts only about 0.05 seconds. Hypokalaemia can cause prolongation of the QT interval, ST-segment depression and T-wave inversion. The opening of the aortic valve occurs during ventricular systole (QRS–T). Isovolumetric contraction also occurs during ventricular systole when the mitral and tricuspid valves are closed (it lasts for 0.05 seconds).

41. D: Hyperventilation

Hyperventilation causes cerebral vasoconstriction due to hypocapnia. Nursing the patient with the head down leads to venous pooling in the cranium and increases intracranial pressure.

System	Parasympathetic		Sympathetic	
	α_1	α_2	β_1	β_2
Heart	↓ rate ↓ atrial contractility ↓ AVN conduction		↑ rate and contractility ↑ AVN conduction ↑ renin secretion	
Vessels	Little effect	Vasoconstriction of arterioles (esp. skin, abdominal viscera and coronary circulation) Constriction of systemic veins		Vasodilatation of coronary arterioles and in skeletal muscles
Bronchus	Bronchoconstriction			Bronchial muscle relaxation
Gut	↑ motility Relaxation of sphincters	↓ motility		↓ motility
Pancreas	↑ exocrine secretion No effect on β cells of islets	↓ exocrine secretion		↑ endocrine secretion by β cells; lipolysis; glycogenolysis; gluconeogenesis
Urogenital	Contraction of detrusor muscles of bladder Relaxation of sphincters	Relaxation of detrusor muscles Contraction of sphincters and pregnant uterus		Relaxation of pregnant uterus
Glands		↓ secretion (lacrimal, salivary, alimentary)		↑ secretion by sweat glands
Eye	Miosis – sphincter pupillae contracts			Mydriasis – dilator pupillae contracts

42. A: Noradrenaline (norepinephrine)

Noradrenaline decreases intestinal secretion. Prostaglandins increase secretion, and are thought to play a major role in thediarrhoea which occurs in inflammatory bowel disease and in radiation enteritis.

43. C: Bile salts act as emulsifying agents

Pancreatic lipase is the most important enzyme in fat digestion. Deficiency of this enzyme may occur as a result of pancreatic disease. Surgical resection of the pancreas leads to steatorrhoea. Pancreatic lipase is more active in the presence of bicarbonate and therefore a low duodenal pH (as seen in gastrinoma) can also lead to steatorrhoea. Lipids and bile salts interact to form micelles. Monoglycerides, cholesterol and fatty acids from the micelles enter the mucosal cells by passive diffusion. The subsequent fate of the fatty acids depends on their size. Fatty acids containing more than 10–12 carbon atoms are re-esterified to triglycerides within the mucosal cells. Chylomicrons containing triglycerides and cholesteryl esters enter the lymphatics and pass into the bloodstream through the thoracic duct. On a moderate fat intake, 95% or more of ingested fat is absorbed.

44. C: If intractable, it may be relieved by lobotomy

Transmission of pain is faster through myelinated fibres (A fibres). The posterior columns relay position-sense, vibration and touch sensations. The spinothalamic tracts relay pain, temperature and light touch. Visceral pain, which is poorly localised, may cuase reflex contraction of nearby muscles. Mu (μ) receptors are opiate receptors which mediate supraspinal analgesia, euphoria, dependence, gut stasis, miosis and depression of respiration. Other surgical procedures used to relieve intractable pain include sympathectomy, myelotomy, posterior rhizotomy, anterolateral cordotomy and thalamotomy.

45. E: Its analogues may be used in the treatment of prostatic carcinoma

LHRH is secreted by the hypothalamus. It stimulates the release of FSH and LH by the anterior pituitary. The release of LHRH is pulsatile. Its analogues have been used recently in the treatment of prostatic and breast cancers, through down-regulation of pituitary receptors, which decreases LH secretion.

46. D: The main receptors in the CTZ are dopaminergic (D_2)

The chemoreceptor trigger zone (CTZ) is located on the lateral walls of the fourth ventricle, outside the blood–brain barrier. Anticholinergic drugs block muscarinic receptors in the vomiting centre and vestibular apparatus (it is the stimulation of these receptors which causes vestibular apparatus-mediated vomiting). $5HT_3$ antagonists (eg ondansetron) are effective in the control of chemotherapy-induced vomiting. Phenothiazines and metoclopramide act mainly on the CTZ. Antihistamines are also useful anti-emetics.

47. C: It has a higher affinity for carbon monoxide than for oxygen

Adult haemoglobin is composed of four haem molecules bound to a single globin molecule, which itself is composed of four polypeptide chains. Haemoglobin can bind CO_2 in a reversible reaction to form carboxyhaemoglobin. Around 30% of CO_2 is carried in the blood in this way. The affinity of the haemoglobin-binding site for CO is around 200 times its affinity for O_2 and the resulting complex is irreversible, so that CO will displace O_2 from oxyhaemoglobin. Hypoxia stimulates haemoglobin production indirectly, via the increased secretion of erythropoietin.

48. A: It may be used to assess the rotation of the heart along its longitudinal axis

The QRS complex is caused by ventricular depolarisation. The cardiac axis is the predominant direction of ventricular depolarisation in the frontal plane. This is commonly determined in the ECG by assessing the mean QRS deflection in leads I and aVF. Ventricular repolarisation is associated with the QT interval. The QRS complex corresponds to the process of isovolumetric contraction, when pressure in the ventricular cavities rises due to the onset of ventricular contraction. The pressure gradient across the atrioventricular valves is reversed, causing closure of the atrioventrcular valve. After closure, the ventricular pressure rises to exceed that in the arteries, when ventricular ejection begins. Tricyclic antidepressant poisoning causes prolongation of the QRS complex. The finding of a large Q wave is always pathological.

49. E: The vital capacity (VC) falls when the patient is moved from an upright to a supine position

In respiratory muscle weakness, the TLC is reduced and the RV is increased due to the reduction in inspiratory and expiratory capacity. This leads to a reduction in VC, but because the FEV_1:VC ratio is normal there is no decrease in FEV_1. Hypercapnia is a late feature. The development of dyspnoea and the fall in VC when lying flat are indicators of bilateral diaphragmatic weakness.

50. B: Prostaglandins

Endothelin is a vasoconstricting peptide synthesised by endothelial cells and by neurones in the paraventricular nucleus of the hypothalamus. Nitric oxide is a potent vasodilator which is synthesised from l-arginine in vessel walls by NO synthases. In addition, inspired NO may be clinically useful as a vasodilator of pulmonary arteries. Iloprost (a prostacyclin PGI_2 analogue) may be beneficial in the treatment of the critically ischaemic limb. Both thromboxane A_2 and adenosine diphosphate cause vasoconstriction. Other factors which cause arteriolar dilatation include decreased sympathetic activity, increased Pco_2, decreased pH and Po_2, lactic acid, histamine, and increased local temperature.

51. D: It suppresses appetite

Leptin is a hormone which is responsible for the regulation of body fat mass. It is a product of the *ob* gene, which is expressed in the placenta and in adipocytes. Its actions generally tend to lead to loss of fat mass and weight. It is secreted by adipocytes and acts on the hypothalamus to suppress appetite and increase metabolism. In obese individuals its levels are very high. This is due to leptin resistance and lack of negative feedback on leptin secretion.

52. E: X is increased in a patient with emphysema

X is the residual volume; Y is the functional residual capacity. TLC is measured using helium dilution. The residual volume is usually increased in emphysema.

53. C: There will be increased atrial naturetic peptide release

There are several normal responses to hypobaria and hypoxia:

1. An increase in ventilation resulting in a respiratory alkalosis
2. An increase in cerebral blood flow
3. An increase in pulmonary artery pressure
4. Changes in carotid body receptor response to neurotransmitters
5. An increase in atrial naturetic peptide from the heart (and a resulting mild diuresis)
6. Endothelial cell damage and alterations in capillary permeability and mediator release.

The climber described has developed acute mountain sickness (AMS), the commonest medical condition occurring at altitude, seen in approximately 40–50% of those who ascend to 14,000 feet or more. It occurs within 8–96 hours of arrival. Slow ascent (no more than 1000 feet a day) and adequate hydration reduce the risk of this occurring. In mild cases AMS resolves with simple analgesia and bedrest, but some climbers only recover when they descend to lower altitudes. Acetazolamide and dexamethasone are also used, both prophylactically and therapeutically.

54. **A: Amyl nitrite will result in a reduced left ventricular outflow tract obstruction**

The left ventricular (LV) outflow tract obstruction in hypertrophic obstructive cardiomyopathy (HOCM) is increased by factors that reduce pre-load and afterload (eg dehydration, sudden adoption of an upright position, nitrates, Valsalva manoevre). Fever and exercise are both positively inotropic, and this also leads to an increase in the outflow tract gradient. Enhanced venous return (eg leg elevation) and increased afterload (squatting, hand-grip) lead to a reduced outflow tract obstruction and improvement in symptoms. Beta-blockers and calcium-channel antagonists are both negatively inotropic and are therefore used in the management of HOCM.

55. **C: The diclofenac has probably caused a drop in cardiac contractility**

The patient is in acute left ventricular failure (LVF), probably secondary to a non-ST-elevation infarct, and this has possibly been exacerbated by the non-steroidal anti-inflammatory drug (NSAID). There will be raised left ventricular end-diastolic pressure and pulmonary capillary pressure (PCP) leading to pulmonary oedema. The reduced cardiac output will result in an increase in systemic vascular resistance (afterload) in an attempt to maintain perfusion pressure. The stroke volume is proportional to the afterload and therefore the high peripheral vascular resistance will lead to a further drop in stroke volume.

In true LVF (as in this case), as opposed to fluid overload, nitrates are a better choice as they will both venodilate (reducing PCP) and vasodilate (reducing afterload), resulting in a net increase in stroke volume and cardiac output. Furosemide (frusemide) will reduce PCP via venodilatation, but it will also result in a reduced cardiac output due to lowered left ventricular end-diastolic pressure.

NSAIDs cause systemic vasoconstriction (via inhibition of prostaglandins, which are up-regulated in heart failure) and therefore reduced cardiac contractility and cardiac output. A lactic acidosis is often seen in LVF, secondary to poor tissue perfusion.

56. A: An increased TLCO

The clinical picture is one of a rapidly progressive glomerulonephritis with pulmonary haemorrhage, most likely to be associated with anti-glomerular basement membrane antibodies (Goodpasture's syndrome). Pulmonary haemorrhage often leads to an acute fall in haemoglobin. The measured diffusion capacity of carbon monoxide (TLCO) is often high in pulmonary haemorrhage, secondary to the presence of haemoglobin in the alveoli. Other causes of a raised TLCO are asthma/bronchitis, hyperkinetic states, left-to-right shunts, polycythaemia and exercise.

57. B: Hypothyroidism

The patient has both symptoms and a biochemical profile consistent with hypothyroidism. A raised prolactin is a well-recognised association. The mechanism of this is not entirely clear but probably involves an increased prolactin response to the rise in thyrotrophin-releasing hormone (TRH). Apart from a pituitary prolactinoma, other pathological causes of a raised prolactin include: hypothalamic/pituitary disease, renal impairment (reduced prolactin excretion) and drugs such as dopamine antagonists (bromocriptine). Physiological causes are sleep, pregnancy, exercise, stress and puberty in girls.

Chapter 7
CLINICAL CHEMISTRY
Questions

1. **Which one of the following is a feature of von Gierke's disease?**

   ☐ A   Hyperlipidaemia
   ☐ B   Autosomal dominant inheritance
   ☐ C   Hepatosplenomegaly and cardiomegaly in infants
   ☐ D   Deficiency of glucose-6-phosphate
   ☐ E   An association with diabetes mellitus

2. **Which one of the following findings is consistent with a diagnosis of untreated phenylketonuria?**

   ☐ A   Cataracts
   ☐ B   Reduced blood phenylalanine level
   ☐ C   Increased pigmentation
   ☐ D   An IQ of 100
   ☐ E   Eczema

3. A 49-year-old businessman is admitted to the Accident and Emergency Department with a one-week history of fever and double vision. A CT scan of his brain shows no abnormalities. A lumbar puncture is performed, which reveals: red blood cells 6 cells/mm^3, white cells 23 cells/mm^3 (90% lymphocytes), total protein 3.2 g/l, glucose 3.0 mmol/l (serum level 5.2 mmol/l), and a low cerebrospinal fluid (CSF) globulin:albumin ratio. Which one of the following diagnoses would be most consistent with the clinical and biochemical findings?

☐ A Neurosyphilis
☐ B Multiple sclerosis (MS)
☐ C Encephalitis
☐ D Cerebral sarcoidosis
☐ E Systemic lupus erythematosus (SLE)

4. A 35-year-old man is brought to the Accident and Emergency Department by the police. He is a regular attender who is known to drink around 30 units of alcohol per day. He is confused and confabulating. Neurological examination shows ataxia and bilateral horizontal nystagmus. Wernicke's encephalopathy is suspected. Which one of the following is also associated with the vitamin deficiency which causes Wernicke's encephalopathy?

☐ A Glossitis
☐ B Reduced blood pyruvate and lactate levels
☐ C Peripheral neuropathy
☐ D An increased incidence in maize eaters
☐ E Narrowing of the pulse pressure

5. Which one of the following may result in a positive Clinitest® reaction?

☐ A Hyperphosphaturia
☐ B Aminoaciduria
☐ C Rifampicin therapy
☐ D Salicylate therapy
☐ E Cystinuria

6. **Which one of the following statements is true of transferrin?**

- [ ] A Its levels are reduced in patients on oral contraceptive therapy
- [ ] B Its levels are reduced in iron deficiency
- [ ] C Its levels are high in haemochromatosis
- [ ] D It is excessively saturated with iron in severe liver disease
- [ ] E It is normally about 70% saturated with iron

7. **In which one of the following conditions would the serum acid phosphatase be elevated?**

- [ ] A Hurler's syndrome
- [ ] B Carcinoma of the rectum
- [ ] C Primary hyperparathyroidism
- [ ] D Gaucher's disease
- [ ] E Vitamin D-resistant rickets

8. **A 16-year-old boy presents to the Accident and Emergency Department with a three-week history of polydipsia and polyuria, visual disturbance and lethargy. His serum glucose is 24 mmol/l and dipstick urinalysis is positive for ketones. An arterial blood gas reveals a pH of 7.24. Which one of the following is the most likely metabolic process occurring in this boy?**

- [ ] A Increased uptake of amino acids
- [ ] B Increased protein catabolism
- [ ] C Increased glucose uptake
- [ ] D Increased lipogenesis
- [ ] E Increased glycogenesis

9. **Which one of the following statements is true regarding free fatty acids?**

- [ ] A Their release is promoted by insulin
- [ ] B They stimulate glycolysis
- [ ] C They are released from adipose tissue during starvation
- [ ] D They are released from adipose tissue when insulin levels are high
- [ ] E They stimulate metabolism via the pentose phosphate pathway

Answers on pages 173–175

10. A 65-year-old man visits his general practitioner complaining of haematuria. Clinical examination is unremarkable and dipstick urinalysis is negative for blood. Which one of the following disorders could potentially explain his symptoms?

- ☐ A Cystinuria
- ☐ B Myoglobinuria
- ☐ C Paroxysmal nocturnal haemoglobinuria
- ☐ D Congenital porphyria
- ☐ E Ethambutol therapy

11. A five-year-old child is investigated by a paediatrician for recent onset of hyperactivity and attention deficit. She also appears to have some loss of co-ordination. A large number of tests are performed, all of which are normal. A more detailed history, however, reveals that the household has recently been decorated, and large quantities of paint were stripped from the walls. Her serum lead level is high at 1.55 μmol/l. Which one of the following may also occur in lead poisoning?

- ☐ A Peripheral oedema
- ☐ B Abdominal pain, relieved by calcium gluconate
- ☐ C Decreased serum iron
- ☐ D Purpura
- ☐ E Diarrhoea

12. A 72-year-old woman attends the Outpatients Clinic complaining of tiredness and lethargy. Her haemoglobin level is 4.3 g/dl. The mean corpuscular volume (MCV) is 112 fl (normal range 80–96 fl); haematinic measurements show a serum vitamin B_{12} level of 66.4 pmol/l (normal range 120–700 pmol/l); serum folate was within the normal range. Which one of the following conditions or drug treatments may have caused this picture?

- ☐ A Phenytoin therapy
- ☐ B Methotrexate therapy
- ☐ C Ulcerative colitis
- ☐ D *Diphyllobothrium latum* infection
- ☐ E *Taenia solium* infection

13. **Which one of the following is a feature of homocystinuria?**

☐ A A high incidence of renal calculi
☐ B An association with dissecting aortic aneurysms
☐ C Upward dislocation of the lens
☐ D Improvement on adopting a cysteine-restricted diet
☐ E Elevated plasma methionine levels

14. **You are called urgently to see a patient on the ward who is fitting. Following an initial assessment, a bedside capillary glucose measurement is taken. The value is 0.9 mmol/l. The patient rapidly returns to normal following the intravenous administration of 25 ml of 50% dextrose. On review of the case notes, it is noted that exactly the same thing has happened several times previously, but the patient is not taking insulin or oral hypoglycaemic agents, and the illicit use of these is not suspected. Which one of the following conditions would explain this clinical picture?**

☐ A Carcinoid syndrome
☐ B Type 2 multiple endocrine neoplasia (MEN 2)
☐ C Hyperthyroidism
☐ D Hypopituitarism
☐ E Acute intermittent porphyria

15. **A 15-year-old girl with a history of acute intermittent porphyria presents to hospital feeling unwell after taking an antibiotic prescribed by her general practitioner. Which one of the following features would most support the suspicion that her symptoms are being caused by an attack of acute intermittent porphyria?**

☐ A Diarrhoea
☐ B Incontinence of urine
☐ C Photosensitive skin rash
☐ D Hypertension
☐ E Increased somnolence

Answers on pages 176–177

16. A 92-year-old lady is admitted from a nursing home. The matron tells you that she has been very constipated for two weeks, and that for the last five days she has become increasingly confused. On examination she is very dehydrated and is twitching. A basic blood screen reveals a corrected serum calcium of 2.99 mmol/l. Which one of the following is the most likely cause?

- [ ] A Thiazide diuretic therapy
- [ ] B Hypothyroidism
- [ ] C Chronic renal failure
- [ ] D Fanconi syndrome
- [ ] E Paget's disease

17. Which one of the following is true of acute intermittent porphyria?

- [ ] A It shows autosomal recessive inheritance
- [ ] B There is skin photosensitivity
- [ ] C Arthritis may occur
- [ ] D Psychosis is common
- [ ] E Peripheral neuropathy is rare

18. Which one of the following is a cause of hypoglycaemia?

- [ ] A Plasmodium malariae infection
- [ ] B Prolactinoma
- [ ] C Hypothyroidism
- [ ] D Glucagonoma
- [ ] E Corticosteroids

19. Which one of the following statements is true regarding iron metabolism?

A   Plasma iron levels follow a circadian rhythm
B   Iron can only cross cell membranes in the ferric form
C   Only 30% of dietary iron is absorbed in the upper small intestine
D   Reduction in gastric acid levels results in increased absorption of iron
E   Turnover of plasma iron is independent of haemopoiesis

20. Which one of the following inhibits hepatic gluconeogenesis?

A   Acidosis
B   Alcohol
C   Insulin
D   Glucagon
E   Corticosteroids

21. Which one of the following conditions can cause proteinuria of more than 15–20 g/day?

A   Amyloidosis
B   Adult Fanconi syndrome
C   Acute renal tubular acidosis
D   Analgesic nephropathy
E   Pelvi-ureteric junction obstruction

22. Which one of the following disorders may cause hypercalcaemia?

A   Systemic sclerosis
B   Hypothyroidism
C   Miliary tuberculosis
D   Myositis ossificans
E   Carcinoid syndrome

23. A 72-year-old man with a history of renal calculi is noted to have a high urinary calcium level. His serum corrected calcium is 2.54 mmol/l. Which one of the following is most likely to explain these findings?

- [ ] A   Multiple myeloma
- [ ] B   Renal tubular acidosis
- [ ] C   Primary hyperparathyroidism
- [ ] D   Hyperthyroidism
- [ ] E   Nutritional rickets

24. A 54-year-old woman with a long-term history of asthma presents to the Respiratory Outpatients Clinic with a history of recurrent attacks of asthma over the last year. She has received multiple courses of corticosteroids from her general practitioner and has not been steroid-free for the last four months. Which one of the following effects is likely to have resulted from her corticosteroid therapy?

- [ ] A   Increased secretion of hydrochloric acid and pepsin
- [ ] B   Reduced protein catabolism
- [ ] C   An increase in intracellular phosphorus
- [ ] D   An increase in the number of circulating lymphocytes
- [ ] E   Decreased urinary calcium

25. A 45-year-old woman has undergone a bilateral adrenalectomy for Cushing's syndrome. Her immediate post-operative course was uneventful, but she has now had several episodes in which she becomes aggressive and confused, and then loses conciousness. These episodes always resolve quickly following the intravenous administration of 50% dextrose. Failure of which one of the following processes is likely to have caused these episodes?

- [ ] A   Protein catabolism
- [ ] B   Gluconeogenesis
- [ ] C   Glycogenolysis
- [ ] D   Glucose absorption from the gut
- [ ] E   Glycogen formation

26. **Which one of the following conditions is characterised by abnormal haem biosynthesis?**

   ☐ A Homozygous thalassaemia
   ☐ B Sickle cell trait
   ☐ C Megaloblastic anaemia
   ☐ D Acute intermittent porphyria
   ☐ E Haemochromatosis

27. **Which one of the following statements is true regarding the uptake of oxygen by haemoglobin?**

   ☐ A It changes iron from the ferric to the ferrous form
   ☐ B It is increased by 2,3-diphosphoglycerate (2,3-DPG)
   ☐ C It is higher in adult haemoglobin than it is in fetal haemoglobin
   ☐ D It increases the buffering capacity of haemoglobin
   ☐ E It is increased in the presence of carboxyhaemoglobin

28. **A 66-year-old man is referred to the Gastroenterology Outpatients Clinic. He has had a basic biochemical screen performed as part of a medical examination for a life insurance policy. All the values were normal apart from a mildly raised alkaline phosphatase of 190 U/l. Which one of the following is most likely to explain these findings?**

   ☐ A Multiple myeloma
   ☐ B Paget's disease
   ☐ C Osteomalacia
   ☐ D Osteoporosis
   ☐ E Metastatic liver malignancy

29. A 41-year-old man has had a total colectomy for Crohn's disease, followed by a further ileal resection after another flare-up. Since the surgery he has been troubled with large-volume diarrhoea attributable to his short bowel. He presents to Casualty complaining of pins and needles and severe muscle cramps in his legs. His serum magnesium is 0.15 mmol/l (normal range 0.75–1.05 mmol/l). Which one of the following also causes these findings?

- [ ] A Hyperthyroidism
- [ ] B Acute renal failure
- [ ] C ACE inhibitors
- [ ] D Idiopathic hypercalcaemia
- [ ] E Chronic dialysis

30. Which one of the following is true of vitamin D?

- [ ] A 1,25-hydroxy-vitamin D production is stimulated by a high circulating phosphate concentration
- [ ] B The enzyme 1α-hydroxylase catalyses the hydroxylation of 25-hydroxycholecalciferol (25(OH)D$_3$) in the kidney
- [ ] C Failure of the initial hydroxylation explains the hypocalcaemia of renal failure
- [ ] D It is hydroxylated to 24,25-dihydroxycholecalciferol (24,25(OH)$_2$D$_3$) in the liver
- [ ] E It is most active in the 25-hydroxycholecalciferol form

31. A 54-year-old woman is admitted to the Accident and Emergency Department unwell, with a metabolic acidosis. Her serum chloride is noted to be 118 mmol/l. Which one of the following would best explain her metabolic disturbance?

- [ ] A Diabetic ketoacidosis
- [ ] B Addison's disease
- [ ] C Vomiting and diarrhoea
- [ ] D Renal tubular acidosis
- [ ] E Overtreatment with diuretics

32. A 58-year-old banker presents to his general practitioner with a history of recurrent painful and swollen knees. There are no other joints involved to date. Which one of the following factors in the history would suggest that his serum uric acid levels may be elevated?

   ☐ A Diabetes mellitus
   ☐ B Hypothyroidism
   ☐ C An elevated serum ferritin
   ☐ D Use of low-dose salicylates
   ☐ E Use of corticosteroids

33. Which one of the following causes an increase in plasma inorganic phosphate?

   ☐ A Gram-negative bacterial septicaemia
   ☐ B Primary hyperparathyroidism
   ☐ C Malignant hyperpyrexia following anaesthesia
   ☐ D Intravenous infusion of isotonic glucose
   ☐ E Vitamin D deficiency

34. A 16-year-old boy presents to the Cardiology Outpatients Clinic with a history of two syncopal attacks during the last six months. He denies having any other symptoms and an echocardiogram arranged by his general practitioner has failed to reveal any structural heart disease. His mother died suddenly of an unknown cause soon after he was born. A 24-hour ambulatory ECG is arranged, during which he has another syncopal attack. The ECG reveals torsades de pointes. Where is the inherited abnormality likely to be?

   ☐ A A bundle of Kent accessory pathway
   ☐ B A mutation in myocardial contractile protein genes
   ☐ C A mutation in potassium channel genes
   ☐ D A mutation in sodium channel genes
   ☐ E A posterior fascicle abnormality

35. A 46-year-old woman is seen by her general practitioner and assessed for risk of ischaemic heart disease. Her total serum cholesterol is 7.2 mmol/l (total:HDL cholesterol ratio 3.2). She is commenced on 40 mg of simvastatin. Ten years later she is admitted to hospital with a suspected myocardial infarction. Measurement at the time reveals a serum total cholesterol of 5.8 mmol/l (total:HDL cholesterol ratio 6.9). Which one of the following may have contributed to the change in HDL cholesterol?

- A   Increasing age
- B   Exercise
- C   A fish diet
- D   Progesterone treatment
- E   Alcohol intake

36. Which one of the following is true regarding cyclooxygenase (COX) enzymes?

- A   COX-1 is not expressed in renal or hepatic vasculature
- B   COX-1 inhibition is responsible for the analgesic effects of non-steroidal anti-inflammatory drugs (NSAIDs)
- C   COX-2 expression is promoted by glucocorticoids
- D   COX-2 mediates vascular homeostasis and platelet aggregation
- E   COX-2 expression is increased in inflammation

37. A 48-year-old woman presents to her general practitioner feeling non-specifically unwell for the last two days. She complains of feeling tired, having occasional chest and joint pains, and has mild dyspnoea. Some routine blood tests are taken, which initially reveal a C-reactive protein of 210 mg/l. With which one of the following conditions is this finding most consistent?

- A   Systemic lupus erythematosus (SLE)
- B   Acute myocardial infarction
- C   Ulcerative colitis
- D   Leukaemia
- E   Viral infection

38. A 32-year-old HIV-positive man attends the Accident and Emergency Department complaining of generalised weakness, back pain and polyuria. In the past he has had chronic hepatitis B infection, for which he received treatment, and iron deficiency anaemia. He has never been on antiretroviral treatment. Serum electrolytes were as follows: Na^+ 150 mmol/l, K^+ 2.8 mmol/l, creatinine 160 µmol/l, phosphate 0.5 mmol/l, corrected Ca^{2+} 1.98 mmol/l. Urinary biochemistry reveals increased urinary loss of potassium, phosphate, calcium, glucose and amino acids. Which one of the following drugs is the likely cause of his recent problems?

   ☐ A Ferrous sulphate
   ☐ B Paracetamol
   ☐ C Ibuprofen
   ☐ D Interferon-α
   ☐ E Adefovir

CLINICAL CHEMISTRY

Answers

1. **A: Hyperlipidaemia**

    Von Gierke's disease is a type 1 glycogen storage disorder in which there is deficiency of glucose-6-phosphatase. Its inheritance is autosomal recessive. It usually presents in infancy with features common to all glycogen storage disorders, namely hepatomegaly, recurrent hypoglycaemia, cardiac failure and muscle weakness. In addition, metabolic acidosis, hyperuricaemia, hyperlipidaemia and ketosis may occur.

2. **E: Eczema**

    Phenylketonuria is an inborn error of amino acid metabolism, with the metabolic fault in the phenylalanine hydroxylase pathway. The diagnosis is made in childhood. The features are eczema, reduced pigmentation, mental retardation (the IQ is usually less than 20) and seizures. A raised blood level of phenylalanine is present from around one week after birth. Early commencement of a low-phenylalanine diet is important.

3. **C: Encephalitis**

    Encephalitis is an inflammatory condition, and is associated with a low CSF globulin:albumin ratio due to leakage of albumin via the blood–brain barrier. The increased ratio seen in MS, SLE, cerebral sarcoidosis and neurosyphilis is due to intrathecal synthesis of immunoglobulin. Cranial nerve palsies may be associated with any of these conditions.

4. C: Peripheral neuropathy

Thiamine is vitamin B_1. Deficiency of this vitamin causes 'dry' beriberi (weight loss and polyneuritis), 'wet' beriberi (high-output cardiac failure) or Wernicke–Korsakoff syndrome. It occurs in individuals whose staple diet is polished rice, and in chronic alcohol abuse. Blood pyruvate is increased, but there is a decrease in red cell transketolase activity and in urinary thiamine excretion. Glossitis is caused by pyridoxine (vitamin B_6) deficiency.

5. D: Salicylate therapy

A positive Clinitest® reaction (the apparent detection of glucose in the urine on dipstick testing) is associated with:

1. Glycosuria – diabetes mellitus, thyrotoxicosis, phaeochromocytoma, post-gastrectomy, severe infection, a lag glucose tolerance curve, pregnancy (reduced renal threshold)
2. Galactosaemia, hereditary fructosaemia, alkaptonuria
3. Drugs – L-dopa, salicylates, vitamin C, isoniazid, tetracyclines.

6. D: It is excessively saturated with iron in severe liver disease

Iron is carried in the plasma in the ferric (Fe^{3+}) form, attached to transferrin. This specific binding protein is normally around one-third saturated with iron. Transferrin levels are raised in pregnancy, iron deficiency anaemia, viral hepatitis, and in patients taking the oral contraceptive pill. Levels are normal or reduced in haemochromatosis.

7. D: Gaucher's disease

Acid phosphatase is found in the prostate gland, platelets, red cells and Gaucher's cells (abnormal reticuloendothelial cells seen in Gaucher's disease). Causes of a raised serum acid phosphatase include metastatic carcinoma of the prostate, Gaucher's disease, myeloid leukaemia, haemolysis, and any metastatic disease with bony involvement. It may also be elevated following rectal examination or the passage of a urinary catheter.

8. B: Increased protein catabolism

The major effects of insulin are:

1. Liver:
   - increased glucose uptake
   - increased glycogen synthesis
   - inhibition of gluconeogenesis
   - increased lipogenesis
   - inhibition of ketogenesis
2. Muscle:
   - increased glucose uptake
   - increased glycogen synthesis
   - increased amino acid uptake
   - increased protein synthesis
   - decreased protein catabolism
3. Adipose tissue:
   - increased glucose entry
   - increased fatty acid synthesis
   - increased lipolysis
   - activation of lipoprotein lipase and hormone-sensitive lipase.

Diabetic ketoacidosis would result in a state of increased protein catabolism.

9. C: They are released from adipose tissue during starvation

The hormone-sensitive lipase (HSL) enzyme is found in adipose tissue. Its action is to hydrolyse triglycerides to produce free fatty acids and glycerol. During fasting, when exogenous glucose is unavailable, endogenous adipose tissue triglyceride is broken down in this way. The free fatty acids and glycerol are transported to the liver and the glycerol enters the gluconeogenic pathway. The resultant glucose is released into the bloodstream at a time when plasma glucose may be falling. HSL is inhibited by insulin. Insulin inhibits the release of free fatty acids from adipose tissue, and a low insulin level is therefore associated with increased release of free fatty acids.

10. D: Congenital porphyria

In porphyria, the porphyrinogens excreted in the urine, δ-aminolaevulinic acid, (δ-ALA) and porphobilinogen (PBG) are colourless, but in ultraviolet light they oxidise to corresponding porphyrins, which are dark red. Myoglobinuria and paroxysmal nocturnal haemoglobinuria would be expected to give a positive urine dipstick test for blood. Rifampicin turns the urine orange-red and ethambutol can result in abnormalities in colour vision.

11. B: Abdominal pain, relieved by calcium gluconate

The clinical features of lead poisoning include abdominal colic, gingivitis (with a blue line on the gums), motor neuropathy and encephalopathy. The haematological effects are numerous and include anaemia, reticulocytosis, basophilic stippling and increased serum iron concentration.

12. D: *Diphyllobothrium latum* infection

Vitamin B_{12} deficiency may occasionally be seen in true vegans due to dietary deficiency. It is more commonly caused by pernicious anaemia and partial/total gastrectomy. Any condition which affects the terminal ileum and its ability to absorb B_{12} may also cause deficiency. These include Crohn's disease, ileal resection, blind-loop syndrome, and infection with the fish tapeworm, *Diphyllobothrium latum*. Phenytoin and methotrexate tend to cause folate deficiency. *Taenia solium*, the pork tapeworm, causes cystercercosis.

13. E: Elevated plasma methionine levels

Homocystinuria is caused by an inborn metabolic block in the conversion of homocystine and serine to cystathionine, due to a deficiency of cystathione β-synthetase. Its clinical features include mental retardation, seizures, osteoporosis, spastic paraplegia, cataracts, downward dislocation of the lens, a high, arched palate, arachnodactyly and recurrent thromboembolic disease, but not dissecting aortic disease. Plasma methionine and urinary homocystine levels are elevated. Treatment is by dietary restriction of methionine and supplementation with cystine.

14. **D: Hypopituitarism**

Spontaneous hypoglycaemia occurs in type 1 and type 3 glycogen storage disorders, Addison's disease and hypopituitarism, galactosaemia, fructose intolerance, leucine sensitivity, alcoholic cirrhosis, post-gastrectomy syndrome, β-cell islet tumours and in hypothyroidism. Islet cell tumours are a feature of the MEN 1 syndrome.

15. **D: Hypertension**

Acute intermittent porphyria shows autosomal dominant inheritance. Clinical features include: fragile skin; gastrointestinal symptoms (abdominal pain, vomiting, constipation); cardiovascular effects (hypertension, tachycardia); and CNS symptoms (peripheral neuropathy, confusion and psychosis). Photosensitivity is a feature of porphyria cutanea tarda.

16. **A: Thiazide diuretic therapy**

Hypercalcaemia can result from:

1. Increased intake/absorption – vitamin D excess, intravenous therapy, sarcoidosis
2. Increased renal reabsorption – thiazide diuretic therapy
3. Increased bone resorption – malignancy (PTH-related peptide or, less commonly, bony metastasis), hyperparathyroidism, thyrotoxicosis, immobilisation
4. Miscellaneous causes – Addison's disease, tuberculosis, phaeochromocytoma, acromegaly.

Chronic renal failure tends to cause hypocalcaemia and hyperphosphataemia.

17. **D: Psychosis is common**

See answer to Question 15.

18. C: Hypothyroidism

See answer to Question 14. *Plasmodium falciparum* infection is most commonly associated with hypoglycaemia, along with treatment with intravenous quinine.

19. A: Plasma iron levels follow a circadian rhythm

Iron is absorbed by an active process in the upper small intestine (approximately 10%) and passes rapidly into the plasma. It can cross membranes only in the ferrous form. Vitamin C, alcohol and gastric acid all increase iron absorption, whereas tetracyclines, phytates, phosphates and gastric achlorhydria reduce it.

20. C: Insulin

Glucagon, cortisol and adrenaline (epinephrine) all stimulate gluconeogenesis. Insulin inhibits gluconeogenesis.

21. A: Amyloidosis

Massive proteinuria is seen in the nephrotic syndrome, which may be the result of diabetes mellitus, systemic lupus erythematosus, inferior vena cava or renal vein thrombosis, or malaria due to *Plasmodium malariae* infection.

22. C: Miliary tuberculosis

See answer to Question 16.

23. B: Renal tubular acidosis

Hypercalciuria may occur in both hypercalcaemia and normocalcaemia:

1. Hypercalciuria with hypercalcaemia:
   – increased bone resorption (primary hyperparathyroidism,

multiple myeloma, malignancy, hyperthyroidism,
immobilisation)
  – increased gut absorption (vitamin D excess, sarcoidosis)
2. Hypercalciuria with normocalcaemia:
  – increased bone resorption (as above, plus osteoporosis,
    Paget's disease, renal tubular acidosis)
  – increased gut absorption (as above, plus idiopathic
    hypercalciuria).

24. A: Increased secretion of hydrochloric acid and pepsin

The actions of glucocorticoids include:

Glycogenesis (liver)
Gluconeogenesis (liver)
Increased protein catabolism
Increased plasma glucose
Lipolysis, free fatty acid mobilisation and oxidation, and increased
ketone production
Anti-inflammatory/anti-allergic properties
Increased resistance to stress
Increased urinary calcium
Increased secretion of hydrochloric acid and pepsin
Decreased lymphocytes and eosinophils; increased neutrophils,
platelets and red cells

25. B: Gluconeogenesis

Hypoglycaemia may occur after adrenalectomy due to the
inhibition of gluconeogenesis. The plasma potassium may fall and
reduced plasma volume may cause hypotension and shock.

26. D: Acute intermittent porphyria

In acute intermittent porphyria there is a defect in the conversion of
porphobilinogen to uroporphyrinogen. Thalassaemia and sickle
cell disease are disorders of globin synthesis.

27. **D: It increases the buffering capacity of haemoglobin**

2,3-DPG binds haemoglobin and stabilises the deoxy form. This reduces the affinity of haemoglobin for oxygen, and causes oxygen release. Oxygen binds to the ferrous form in haem to form oxyhaemoglobin. In both myoglobin and haemoglobin, the iron of the haem group is in the ferrous form. When in the ferric (Fe^{3+}) form, the proteins are methaemoglobin and metmyoglobin. The oxygen affinity is increased in cells containing fetal haemoglobin and with methaemoglobin and carboxyhaemoglobin, leading to tissue hypoxia.

28. **B: Paget's disease**

Serum alkaline phosphatase is raised in growing children, pregnancy, liver disease (eg obstructive jaundice, cirrhosis, malignancy) and in bone disease involving an increased metabolic turnover of bone (eg Paget's disease, osteomalacia, metastatic disease, hyperparathyroidism). Myeloma and osteomalacia would usually result in changes to serum calcium levels as well and liver metastases would be expected to cause derangements in more than one liver enzyme.

29. **E: Chronic dialysis**

The causes of hypomagnesaemia include: severe diarrhoea, chronic dialysis, diuretic therapy, acute pancreatitis, chronic alcoholism, malabsorption and fistulae.

30. **B: The enzyme 1α-hydroxylase catalyses the hydroxylation of 25-hydroxycholecalciferol (25(OH)D₃) in the kidney**

Cholecalciferol (vitamin D_3) is hydroxylated, first in the liver to produce 25-hydroxycholecalciferol (25(OH)D_3) and next in the kidney to form both 1,25(OH)$_2$$D_3$ and 24,25(OH)$_2$$D_3$. The prinicipal circulating form is 25-hydroxycholecalciferol, but further hydroxylation is needed to confer biological activity. Production of 1,25(OH)$_2$$D_3$ is stimulated by a low circulating phosphate, and by high levels of circulating parathyroid hormone (PTH), oestrogen, prolactin and growth hormone.

31. D: Renal tubular acidosis

Hyperchloraemic acidosis is often associated with hypokalaemia. It occurs when bicarbonate is lost in a one-to-one exchange for chloride. Causes include ureterosigmoidostomy, renal tubular acidosis, acetazolamide treatment and hyperventilation. Hypochloraemic acidosis can be caused by loss of gastrointestinal fluids, overtreatment with diuretics, chronic respiratory acidosis, diabetic ketoacidosis or adrenal insufficiency.

32. D: Use of low-dose salicylates

Hyperuricaemia is caused by:

1. Increased purine synthesis – primary gout, Lesch–Nyhan syndrome
2. Increased purine turnover – myelo- and lymphoproliferative disorders, polycythaemia, severe exfoliative psoriasis
3. Decreased excretion of uric acid – primary gout, renal failure, diabetic ketoacidosis
4. Drugs – thiazide and loop diuretics, pyrazinamide, salicylate in low doses, cytotoxics and alcohol.

33. C: Malignant hyperpyrexia following anaesthesia

During carbohydrate utilisation, phosphate and potassium enter the cells with glucose. Intravenous glucose infusion may cause severe hypophosphataemia, and blood for measurement of inorganic phosphate should therefore be taken from fasting patients. If rapid separation of plasma from red blood cells is not achieved, erythrocyte phosphates and inorganic phosphates will result in the recording of a falsely high concentration of serum phosphates. Parathyroid hormone causes phosphaturia and a reduced plasma phosphate. Septicaemia also causes hypophosphataemia.

34. C: A mutation in potassium channel genes

The diagnosis is likely to be congenital long QT syndrome, a voltage-gated ion channel defect affecting the cardiac potassium channels. The Brugada syndrome is another cause of sudden cardiac death in the absence of structural heart disease and is thought to be due to mutations in sodium channel genes. Drugs, hormones, growth factors and metabolites interact with cell receptors and stimulate second-messenger systems to produce changes in the state of cells. Examples of ion channel disorders include:

1. Ligand-gated ion channel disorders – cystic fibrosis (ATP-gated chloride channel), nocturnal frontal lobe epilepsy (neuronal nicotinic acetylcholine receptor) and startle disease (glycine receptor)
2. Voltage-gated ion channel disorders – long QT syndrome (cardiac potassium channels), myotonia congenita (skeletal muscle chloride channel), hyperkalaemic periodic paralysis (skeletal muscle sodium channel), hypokalaemic periodic paralysis (skeletal muscle calcium channel).

35. D: Progesterone treatment

High levels of high-density lipoprotein (HDL) cholesterol are thought to be protective against coronary heart disease. It has been suggested that a high total:HDL cholesterol ratio is of greater value in predicting risk than a high total cholesterol or a high low-density lipoprotein (LDL) cholesterol. Causes of a raised HDL cholesterol include increasing age, exercise, a fish diet and moderate alcohol consumption. Causes of a reduced HDL include smoking, obesity, a high-carbohydrate diet, and therapy with androgens or progesterones. A number of rare genetic disorders, such as Tangier disease, familial HDL deficiency, familial hypoalphalipoproteinaemia and lipoprotein lipase deficiency also result in a low serum HDL.

36. E: COX-2 expression is increased in inflammation

Cyclooxygenase (COX) exists in two isoforms, COX-1 and COX-2. COX-1 is expressed in most tissues and is involved in many regulatory processes, such as gastric cytoprotection, vascular homeostasis, platelet aggregation and kidney function. Most adverse effects of NSAIDs are caused by COX-1 inhibition. COX-2 is undetectable in most tissues and shows increased expression in states of inflammation. Its expression in fibroblasts is promoted by interleukin-1 (IL-1) and growth factors and inhibited by glucocorticoids. COX-2 produces the prostanoids involved in inflammatory responses. The analgesic effects of NSAIDs are due to COX-2 inhibition.

37. B: Acute myocardial infarction

C-reactive protein (CRP) is an acute phase protein produced by the liver which is raised following trauma, infection, malignancy or autoimmune disease. Other examples of acute phase proteins include: serum amyloid precursor, α_1-antitrypsin, fibrinogen, haptoglobin and complement. A marked rise in the CRP is seen in connective tissue disorders (except SLE), malignancy, bacterial infection, necrosis (eg acute myocardial infarction), Crohn's disease and trauma (including surgery). A mild increase may be seen in viral infection, ulcerative colitis, SLE and with the use of steroids. The CRP is frequently not raised in SLE (unless there is superadded infection), ulcerative colitis, leukaemia, pregnancy, anaemia, polycythaemia and heart failure.

38. E: Adefovir

The patient has an aquired form of Fanconi syndrome. This is characterised by a renal tubular defect, with urinary loss of potassium, phosphate, calcium, magnesium, amino acids and glucose, as well as a proximal renal tubular acidosis. Symptoms are related to low serum levels of these electrolytes, acidosis and osteomalacia. The condition may be inherited or acquired:

1. Inherited causes include: cystinosis, galactosaemia, hereditary fructose intolerance, type 1 glycogen storage disease and Wilson's disease
2. Acquired causes:
    - poisons – mercury, lead, zinc, bismuth, arsenic, paraquat
    - drugs – salicylates, cisplatin, adefovir
    - renal disease – acute tubular necrosis, nephrotic syndrome, renal graft rejection
    - nutritional deficiency – vitamin B_{12} deficiency, vitamin D deficiency, kwashiorkor.

Chapter 8

STATISTICS AND EPIDEMIOLOGY

Questions

1. **Which one of the following statements is true?**

   ☐ A   Logarithmic scales measure absolute changes in a variable
   ☐ B   A log-normal distribution is a skewed distribution when graphed using a logarithmic scale
   ☐ C   In distributions which are markedly skewed, the geometic mean is a more appropriate measure than the arithmetic mean
   ☐ D   The mode is the midpoint in a frequency distribution curve
   ☐ E   In a positively skewed distribution, the median is greater than the mode, but greater than the mean

2. **Which one of the following statements is true?**

   ☐ A   The standard error of the mean (SEM) is generally larger than the standard deviation (SD)
   ☐ B   The standard error of the mean provides a measure of the spread of observations around the mean
   ☐ C $SD = \dfrac{SEM}{\sqrt{n}}$
   ☐ D   The mean and standard deviation of a random sample will generally be different from the mean and standard deviation of the population
   ☐ E   The coefficient of variation is derived from the range

Answers on page 193

3. In a hypertension screening programme in which 1550 men aged 30–69 years have been examined, both the mean and the median of the diastolic blood pressure distribution are approximately 83 mmHg and the standard deviation is 12 mmHg. Which one of the following statements is true?

- A Approximately 99% of the men have diastolic blood pressures between 59 mmHg and 107 mmHg
- B The distribution is skewed
- C 95% of observations fall within two standard errors of the mean
- D The range 59–107 mmHg will include the mean of all screened men with a 95% probability
- E 55 of the men will have a diastolic blood pressure greater than 107 mmHg

4. Which one of the following statements regarding the chi-squared test is true?

- A It is used as an alternative to the t-test to determine the difference between two means
- B It can be used to test the difference between two nominal variables
- C The smaller the value of the chi-squared value, the more likely it is to be significant
- D The number of degrees of freedom of the test for a two-by-two table is 2
- E It assumes that all table cells have an expected frequency > 5

5. The correlation coefficient (r) between two variables is estimated from a sample of pairs of observations. Which of the following statements is true?

- A If $r = 0.1$, there is unlikely to be a significant relationship between the two variables
- B If $r = 0.3$ with $P < 0.005$, then there is a strong and statistically significant correlation between the two variables
- C It indicates by how much each variable changes when the other changes
- D If $r = 0.9$, there is a good negative correlation between the two variables
- E It expresses the proportion of the variance of each variable that is explained by its linear relationship with the other

6. **Which one of the following statements about retrospective and prospective studies is true?**

☐ A   In a prospective study the cohort originally selected consists of people who are found to have the disease

☐ B   Prospective studies allow direct determination of incidence rates

☐ C   A retrospective study involves a survey of the prevalence of the disease in different strata of the population

☐ D   The retrospective approach has the advantage that there is little or no bias in the assessment of exposure to the suspected factor

☐ E   The prospective approach may be used to determine the aetiology of a rare disease

7. **The table below shows the results from a screening test for diabetes used on 10,000 people (Test A). The cut-off glucose level used was 8 mmol/l or above.**

Screening test result	True diagnosis		
	Diabetic	Non-diabetic	Total
Positive	34	20	54
Negative	116	9830	9946
Total	150	9850	10,000

In Test B, the screening cut-off level was lowered to glucose levels of 6 mmol/l or above. Which one of the following is correct?

☐ A   The sensitivity of Test A is 22.6%

☐ B   The specificity of Test A is 75%

☐ C   The specificity of Test B would be greater than that of Test A

☐ D   The number of false positives would be greater with Test A than with Test B

☐ E   Initial screening provides an incidence estimate and subsequent screenings, a prevalence estimate

Answers on pages 194–196

8. **Which one of the following statements regarding confidence intervals (CI), around a measurement is true?**

    ☐ A The lower and upper boundaries of a CI may indicate important treatment effect in negative trials
    ☐ B They are calculated from the mean and the standard deviation
    ☐ C A 99% CI will be narrower than the corresponding 95% CI
    ☐ D The width of the CI increases with sample size
    ☐ E 99% of observations lie within 2 standard deviations of the mean

9. **In a study of 100 HIV-infected patients before the availability of effective antiretroviral treatment, the distribution of time from AIDS diagnosis to death was positively skewed, with a peak at two years and a median survival of three years. Which one of the following statements is true?**

    ☐ A More than half the patients were dead by three years
    ☐ B The mean survival will be greater than the median survival
    ☐ C Most patients died later rather than earlier
    ☐ D The 50th and 51st patients in the study died at three years
    ☐ E The mean survival is less than three years

10. **In a study of patients with seizures, 50 patients had an electroencephalogram (EEG) performed, of which 30 were abnormal. Ten per cent of normal people have EEG abnormalities. Which one of the following statements is true?**

    ☐ A The specificity is 60%
    ☐ B The sensitivity is 90%
    ☐ C The sensitivity of the EEG in detecting seizures depends on the prevalence of seizures
    ☐ D The positive predictive value is 50%
    ☐ E If the prevalence of seizures in the population is 5%, and 1000 people are to be screened in a month, the number of true positives will be 30

11. **Which one of the following statistical tests requires a normal population distribution?**

☐ A Wilcoxon rank sum test
☐ B Spearman's rank correlation
☐ C Chi-squared test
☐ D Variance estimation
☐ E Mann–Whitney U test

12. **Two variables, X and Y, are studied for a population and the simple correlation coefficient (r) is equal to +0.8. This correlation coefficient indicates which one of the following?**

☐ A Variable X and variable Y have the same unit of measure
☐ B Variable X and variable Y are causally related
☐ C There is an inverse linear relationship between variable X and variable Y
☐ D Variable X and variable Y are strongly associated
☐ E A unit increase in variable X is associated with a corresponding increase by 0.8 in variable Y

13. **The prevalence of tuberculosis continues to rise in the UK. Which one of the following statements about the period prevalence of tuberculosis in 2004 is correct?**

☐ A It measures the number of existing cases but not new incident cases in 2004
☐ B It is independent of the duration of the illness
☐ C It is independent of the incidence of tuberculosis
☐ D It measures the number of people with tuberculosis at a random single time point in 2004
☐ E It can be estimated from a cross-sectional study

14. **Which one of the following statements about a type 1 error is true?**

☐ A   It is the acceptance of a null hypothesis that is actually true
☐ B   It is often assigned a value of 0.5 in studies
☐ C   It is also called the 'β error'
☐ D   It is used to help determine an appropriate sample size for a study
☐ E   It is equal to 1 minus the β error

15. **In a proposed clinical trial of a new anti-hypertensive drug, which one of the following would require an increase in the sample size?**

☐ A   A decrease in the specified power of the study
☐ B   An increase in the significance level from 1% to 5%
☐ C   An increase in the difference in the blood pressure reduction to be detected
☐ D   A decrease in the type 2 error rate
☐ E   A decrease in the standard deviation of blood pressure measurements

16. **A suspected causative factor of a disease is to be investigated. Which one of the following is a weakness of a case–control study compared to a prospective study in studies of causation?**

☐ A   They are costly and take longer
☐ B   There may be bias in determining the presence or absence of a suspected causal factor
☐ C   There may be bias in determining the presence or absence of the resulting disease
☐ D   It is more difficult to obtain controls
☐ E   It is more difficult to ensure comparability of cases and controls

17. **Controls are needed in a retrospective case–control study because of which one of the following?**

- ☐ A They are matched to the cases for suspected aetiological factors
- ☐ B They may be followed up in order to determine whether they develop the disease in question
- ☐ C They increase the sample size, so that statistical significance may be achieved
- ☐ D They allow evaluation of whether or not the frequency of a characteristic or past exposure among the cases is different from the frequency of these features among comparable people in the population who are free of the disease
- ☐ E They allow a comparison of disease rates across study groups

18. **In a randomised trial of captopril versus placebo in patients with acute myocardial infarction, and a left ejection function <40%, the mortality was 0.20 in the captopril arm and 0.25 in the placebo arm. Which one of the following represents the numbers needed to treat with captopril to prevent one death?**

- ☐ A 1/(0.20/0.25)
- ☐ B 1–(0.20–0.25)
- ☐ C 1/0.20
- ☐ D 0.20–0.25/0.25
- ☐ E 1/(0.20–0.25)

19. **Which one of the following rates are correctly matched with the appropriate application?**

- ☐ A Crude rate – used to compare events in different populations
- ☐ B Direct age-adjusted rate – commonly used for epidemic investigations of acute diseases
- ☐ C Age-specific rate – used to compare disease rates in different populations
- ☐ D Incidence rate – used as a measure of the burden of disease in a population
- ☐ E Prevalence rate – diseases of long duration are less well represented in prevalence surveys

STATISTICS AND EPIDEMIOLOGY

Answers

1. **C: In distributions which are markedly skewed, the geometic mean is a more appropriate measure than the arithmetic mean**

   On an arithmetic scale, equal distances measure equal absolute distances, while on a logarithmic scale, equal distances measure equal proportional distances (ie percentage changes in a variable). A log-normal distribution is a skewed distribution when graphed using an arithmetic scale, but is a normal distribution when graphed using a logarithmic scale. The geometric mean is used as a substitute for the arithmetic mean when the distribution is skewed. It is the anti-log of a mean calculated from observations which have been transformed to a log scale. The mode is the most commonly occurring value in a series of values and is therefore the maximum point in a frequency distribution curve. It is useful in practical epidemiological work, such as for determining the peak disease occurrence in the investigation of a disease outbreak.

2. **D: The mean and standard deviation of a random sample will generally be different from the mean and standard deviation of the population**

   The standard error (SE) measures the variability of a sample statistic (ie mean or proportion) in relation to the true population characteristic (ie how accurate the sample mean is as an estimate of the population mean). The SEM is generally smaller than the standard deviation (SD). The standard deviation is the measure of the variability of the observations:

$$\text{Standard error} = \frac{\text{Standard deviation of observations in a sample}}{\sqrt{\text{Sample size}}}$$

$$\text{The coefficient of variation (\%)} = \frac{\text{SD}}{\text{Mean}} \times 100$$

3. **D: The range 59–107 mmHg will include the mean of all screened men with a 95% probability**

   The distribution of diastolic blood pressure is normal or Gaussian, because the mean and median values are equal. Therefore, 95% of observations fall within two standard deviations (not standard errors) of the mean (ie between 59 and 107 mmHg). Only 2.5% of the men will have a diastolic blood pressure greater than 107 mmHg.

4. **B: It can be used to test the difference between two nominal variables**

   The chi-squared test is used to determine the difference between observed and expected frequencies or between two or more frequencies. The calculated chi-squared value (χ^2) is compared with a critical value of χ^2 from tables, at a predetermined significance level and appropriate degrees of freedom. The larger the χ^2 value, the smaller the probability P, and the more likely it is that the null hypothesis is untrue. The statistical significance of the results also depends on the size of the table, represented by the degrees of freedom (df). The number of degrees of freedom for a two-by-two table is 1 ie (2 columns–1) × (2 rows–1). The assumptions for the test are: independence of observations; at least 80% of the cells with expected frequencies greater than five; and all cells with expected frequencies greater than one.

5.   **A: If r = 0.1, there is unlikely to be a significant relationship between the two variables**

The correlation coefficient (r) describes the strength of the linear relationship between the two variables. Its value can range from -1 (high negative correlation) to $+1$ (high positive correlation).

Correlation coefficient (r)	Degree of association
0.8 to 1.0	Strong
0.5 to 0.8	Moderate
0.2 to 0.5	Weak
0 to 0.2	Negligible

r may be strong but statistically insignificant because of a small sample size and vice versa. The regression coefficient, but *not* the correlation coefficient indicates how much each variable changes when the other changes. r^2 expresses the proportion of the variance of each variable that is explained by its linear relationship with the other.

6.   **B: Prospective studies allow direct determination of incidence rates**

In a prospective cohort study, exposed and non-exposed patients are identified and followed over time to determine the incidence of a specific clinical disease or event. For example, a population of smokers and non-smokers are followed up to provide comparison rates for lung cancer or heart disease. Cross-sectional studies provide information on disease prevalence in a population. Case–control (retrospective) studies compare individuals with and without a disease to determine possible associations or risk factors for the disease in question. Bias may influence the recall of exposure in these studies if possible associations are known, such as the association between cigarette smoking and lung cancer. A case–control study is relatively easy and inexpensive to conduct because long-term follow-up is not required, and this type of study is therefore suitable for studying rare diseases.

7. **A: The sensitivity of test A is 22.6%**

    The **sensitivity** of a screening test is the test's ability to correctly identify those individuals who have diabetes:

    $$= \frac{a}{a + c} \times 100 = \frac{34}{34 + 116} = \frac{34}{150} = 22.67\%$$

    The **specificity** is the test's ability to identify correctly those individuals who do not have the disease:

    $$= \frac{d}{b + d} \times 100 = \frac{9830}{20 + 9830} = \frac{9830}{9850} = 99.8\%$$

    Lowering the screening cut-off level increases the sensitivity and lowers the number of false positives, and decreases the specificity and number of false negatives. The first time that screening is carried out is called the 'prevalence screen', because cases of diabetes will have been present for varying lengths of time. During the second round of screening, most cases will have had their onset between the first and second screening. Second and subsequent screenings are therefore called 'incidence screens'.

8. **A: The lower and upper boundaries of a CI may indicate important treatment effects in negative trials**

    In a normal distribution approximately 68% of the observations fall within one standard deviation of the mean and 99% fall within 2.6 standard deviations of the mean. A 99% CI will be wider than the corresponding 95% CI. The width of the CI also depends on the sample size – larger samples produce narrower CIs.

9. **D: The 50th and 51st patients in the study died at three years**

    In a positively skewed distribution, the mean will be greater than the median, which in turn will be greater than the mode.

10. **E:** **If the prevalence of seizures in the population is 5%, and 1000 people are to be screened in a month, the number of true positives will be 30**

EEG test result	True diagnosis	
	Seizures	No seizures
Positive	30	10
Negative	20	90
Total	50	100

Sensitivity = 30/50 × 100 = 60%; specificity = 90/100 × 100 = 90%.

The sensitivity and specificity are independent of the disease prevalence in the population being tested. The low sensitivity implies an unacceptably high false-negative rate for a serious condition such as seizures.

The **positive predictive value** is a test's ability to identify those people who truly have the disease from among all those whose screening tests are positive. In this example the positive predictive value is 75% – the number of people with disease who tested positive (30) divided by the total number of people who tested positive (40).

Out of 1000 people screened, 50 will have the disease, a prevalence of 5%. Now a + c = 50 and with a sensitivity of 60%, this means that a = 30 and c = 20 (false negatives). Now b + d = 950, with a specificity of 90%, making d = 855 and b (false positives) = 95.

11. **D:** **Variance estimation**

Non-parametric tests make no assumptions about the underlying distribution of the sample. Parametric tests assume that the population is normally distributed, and that the variance of the samples is the same. Spearman's and Kendall's rank correlation coefficients are the non-parametric alternatives to Pearson's correlation coefficient.

12. D: Variable X and variable Y are strongly associated

The **correlation coefficient** is used to indicate the extent to which two variables change with one another in a linear manner. The two variables can have the same or different units of measure, but the correlation coefficient is unitless. A –1 value indicates a strong inverse linear relationship (an increase in one variable is associated with a decrease in the other) while +1 indicates a strong direct linear association. Causality cannot be determined from the correlation coefficient, because the two variables may be associated through a third variable rather than directly.

13. E: It can be estimated from a cross-sectional study

The period **prevalence** is the number of cases, old and new, of a specified disease during a specified time period, divided by the estimated mid-interval population at risk. Since the prevalence includes all cases in the community, it is determined by both the incidence and the duration of the disease process. There are two kinds of prevalence. Point prevalence is measured at a single point in time; period prevalence is the number of cases that were present at any time during a defined period of time.

14. D: It is used to help determine an appropriate sample size for a study

A type 1 error, or α error, is the rejection of the null hypothesis when it is actually true. Type 1 error is used to help determine the sample size of a study and to test the null hypothesis, which is often rejected at the arbitrary cut-off of 5% probability due to chance. The β error is the acceptance as true of a false null hypothesis, and the formula '1 minus the β error' is used to calculate the power of the study.

15. D: A decrease in the type 2 error rate

The determinants of sample size include the size of difference in outcome between groups; the probability of a type 1 error (ie false positive results where the significance level = type 1 error (usually 0.05 or 5%)); the probability of a type 2 error (ie false negative result, where power required = 1–type 2 error (usually 0.8 or 80%)); the variability of observations; and proportion of patients experiencing outcome of interest.

16. B: There may be bias in determining the presence or absence of a suspected causal factor

Although time-consuming, a cohort study allows for determination of a population-based rate of the event under question. A case–control study, on the other hand, is relatively easy and inexpensive to conduct because long-term follow-up is not required. In a cohort study, potential bias is lessened because exposure can be determined prior to the onset of disease. The incidence of an event or disease for exposed and non-exposed populations can be calculated for a cohort study but not in a case–control study. Causality cannot be determined for either case–control study.

17. D: They allow evaluation of whether or not the frequency of a characteristic or past exposure among the cases is different from the frequency of these features among comparable people in the population who are free of the disease

See explanation to Question 16.

18. E: 1/(0.20–0.25)

The number needed to treat (NNT) is the inverse of the absolute risk reduction (ARR). It represents the number of patients who need to be treated to prevent one death.

19. C: Age-specific rate – used to compare disease rates in different populations

Crude rates are summary rates for an entire population. They are easy to calculate because only the number of events and the total population are required. They cannot, however, be used to compare events in different populations because the rate depends on the age-sex composition of the total population.

Adjusted rates are summary rates for the total population, but they are fictitious. By using a standard population or standard age-specific rates, they equalise the differences in the population at risk so that the rates are comparable. Adjusted rates are difficult to calculate because the demographic composition of the population must be known. They are frequently used to compare birth and death rates in different populations. They are seldom used for epidemic investigations of acute diseases.

Age-specific rates are calculated for various strata of the population. Although they are difficult to calculate because more information about the demographic composition of the community must be known than for the other rates, they can be used to compare events in similar age groups in different populations.

Prevalence measures the burden of disease in a population. The **incidence** is the number of new cases of a specified disease occurring during a specific time interval divided by the total population at risk during the same time interval. These rates are used in epidemic investigations using a particular population which is observed for a limited period of time.

Chapter 9

PHARMACOLOGY

Questions

1. A 27-year-old woman is four weeks post-partum. She is breastfeeding. She has heard that some drugs are dangerous for her to take as they can be passed to the baby in her milk. Which one of the following drugs is contraindicated in breastfeeding mothers?

    ☐ A   Warfarin
    ☐ B   Insulin
    ☐ C   Lithium
    ☐ D   Propylthiouracil
    ☐ E   Benzylpenicillin

2. A patient is on the Intensive Care Unit with multi-organ failure of unknown origin. The Microbiology Department informs you that a Gram-negative organism has grown from her blood cultures, and they have advised starting treatment with gentamicin. Which one of the following is true of this class of antibiotics?

    ☐ A   They are metabolised extensively in the liver
    ☐ B   They accumulate in tissues as treatment progresses
    ☐ C   The risk of ototoxicity increases when they are given with ACE inhibitors
    ☐ D   A tendency to ototoxicity can be inherited in nuclear DNA
    ☐ E   They are effective treatment for infection with *Streptococcus pneumoniae*

Answers on page 219

3. A 32-year-old lady is seen by the medical registrar on call with a blood pressure of 170/130 mmHg. She is 34 weeks' pregnant and has had no problems in her pregnancy so far. Dipstick urinalysis reveals protein +. Which one of the following drugs is contraindicated in controlling her blood pressure?

☐ A Hydralazine
☐ B Methyldopa
☐ C Nifedipine
☐ D Enalapril
☐ E Labetolol

4. A 65-year-old diabetic is known to have chronic renal impairment, with a baseline creatinine of 170 μmol/l. He presents with peripheral oedema and mild breathlessness. He also appears to have cellulitis affecting his right leg. There are several agents you may wish to use in his treatment. The dose of which one of the following should be reduced in this patient?

☐ A Erythromycin
☐ B Metronidazole
☐ C Furosemide (frusemide)
☐ D Meropenem
☐ E Rifampicin

5. A 72-year-old man is admitted from his nursing home with a two-week history of profuse diarrhoea. There is no history of abdominal pain or vomiting. A drug-related cause is suspected. Which one of the following drugs is the likely cause?

☐ A Amitriptyline
☐ B Ramipril
☐ C Disopyramide
☐ D Magnesium trisilicate
☐ E Colestyramine

6. A 54-year-old woman presents following a collapse. She is mildly confused. On examination, she has marked postural hypotension. Her serum sodium is 161 mmol/l. She claims to have been passing larger volumes of urine over the last week. Which one of the following drugs is the likely cause?

- [ ] A Desmopressin
- [ ] B Sodium valproate
- [ ] C Carbamazepine
- [ ] D Cyclophosphamide
- [ ] E Lithium

7. Which one of the following drugs avoids hepatic first-pass metabolism?

- [ ] A Ethinylestradiol
- [ ] B Propranolol
- [ ] C Colestyramine
- [ ] D Enalapril
- [ ] E Isosorbide dinitrate

8. A 70-year-old man has type 2 diabetes that is normally well controlled on an oral sulphonylurea. He presents with an episode of hypoglycaemia. No obvious precipitating factor can be found, but he tells you that his general practitioner recently started him on a new tablet. Which one of the following drugs would account for his symptoms?

- [ ] A Lithium
- [ ] B Co-trimoxazole
- [ ] C Rifampicin
- [ ] D Bendroflumethiazide (bendrofluazide)
- [ ] E Phenytoin

Answers on pages 219–221

9. A 46-year-old man with type 2 diabetes is seen by his general practitioner for assessment of further risk factors for coronary artery disease. His serum cholesterol is 4.5 mmol/l and triglycerides 1.2 mmol/l. Two years later, he has a repeat sample taken, which reveals a total cholesterol of 5.6 mmol/l and triglyceride concentration of 4.5 mmol/l. Which one of the following drugs may have caused the raised fasting serum triglyceride concentration?

- [ ] A Nifedipine
- [ ] B Gliclazide
- [ ] C Colestyramine
- [ ] D Captopril
- [ ] E Clopidogrel

10. A 31-year-old man is newly diagnosed with HIV infection. His current CD4 count is 43 cells/mm³. He is due to be started on an antiretroviral regime containing zidovudine. Which one of the following is true of zidovudine?

- [ ] A It blocks the viral protease enzyme
- [ ] B It is contraindicated in severe neutropenia
- [ ] C It is a structural analogue of guanidine
- [ ] D It has a half-life of 12 hours
- [ ] E It is usually given once a day

11. Which one of the following drugs is safe in patients with acute intermittent porphyria?

- [ ] A Chlorpromazine
- [ ] B Chlorpropamide
- [ ] C Phenytoin
- [ ] D Rifampicin
- [ ] E Erythromycin

12. A 64-year-old man with type 2 diabetes is admitted with central crushing chest pain. An electrocardiogram (ECG) reveals inferolateral ischaemic changes and he is commenced immediately on aspirin. Aspirin will potentiate the action of which one of the following drugs?

☐ A Penicillin V
☐ B Chlorpropramide
☐ C Temazepam
☐ D Ramipril
☐ E Insulin

13. A 24-year-old woman is admitted to hospital with sepsis secondary to severe left leg cellulitis. She is treated with various antibiotics and makes a gradual recovery. On day 6 of her admission, the medical house officer notices that her serum creatinine has been rising steadily and is now 241 μmol/l. Which one of the following drugs would be safe to continue?

☐ A Gentamicin
☐ B Oxytetracycline
☐ C Flucloxacillin
☐ D Amoxicillin
☐ E Erythromycin

14. Which one of the following is safe in patients on monoamine-oxidase-inhibitor therapy?

☐ A Pethidine
☐ B Co-trimoxazole
☐ C Coffee
☐ D Imipramine
☐ E L-dopa

15. A 17-year-old girl sees her general practitioner, complaining of a florid rash over her face, arms and legs, which started while she was on holiday in Spain. She was recently prescribed a drug that the doctor suspects may be the cause. Which one of the following medications is the most likely cause of her photosensitivity?

☐ A Doxycycline
☐ B Erythromycin
☐ C Phenytoin
☐ D Nifedipine
☐ E Diazepam

16. The simultaneous administration of which one of the following pairs of drugs is safe?

☐ A Oral contraceptives and rifampicin
☐ B Warfarin and chloral hydrate
☐ C Digoxin and erythromycin
☐ D L-dopa and phenelzine
☐ E Digoxin and propranolol

17. A 38-year-old woman presents to the Accident and Emergency Department with a one-week history of worsening jaundice. Her liver function tests are as follows: bilirubin 56 mmol/l, aspartate aminotransferase (AST) 1110 U/l, alanine aminotransferase (ALT) 986 U/l, alkaline phosphatase (ALP) 67 U/l and γ-glutamyl transferase (GGT) 200 U/l. Which one of the following drugs is the most likely cause of her abnormal biochemistry?

☐ A Amitriptyline
☐ B Glibenclamide
☐ C Halothane
☐ D Oral contraceptive pill
☐ E Norethandrolone

18. A 78-year-old woman is brought into Casualty fitting. Prior to her seizure, her husband noticed that she couldn't use her left arm, and that her speech was slurred. Despite doses of rectal and intravenous diazepam, she continues to fit. It is decided to treat her with intravenous phenytoin. Which one of the following is true regarding treatment with phenytoin?

- [ ] A   A loading dose is not needed to achieve a rapid effect
- [ ] B   Toxicity is associated with a macrocytic anaemia
- [ ] C   Protein-bound iodine is increased
- [ ] D   Toxicity is associated with sensorineural hearing loss
- [ ] E   After a steady state is reached, doubling the dose will approximately double the plasma concentration

19. Which one of the following drugs has a relatively broad therapeutic window?

- [ ] A   Lithium
- [ ] B   Gentamicin
- [ ] C   Cyclophosphamide
- [ ] D   Aminophylline
- [ ] E   Amiodarone

20. A 32-year-old woman from the Ivory Coast is admitted with a history of fever, headache and seizures. She has a past history of epilepsy and is on sodium valproate. She receives a loading dose of intravenous phenytoin and a lumbar puncture is performed. A diagnosis of tuberculous meningitis is made. She is commenced on quadruple antituberculous therapy and makes a good recovery. She attends the Outpatients Clinic two months later, when she informs you that she is three weeks' pregnant. Which one of the following drugs would be safe to continue?

- [ ] A   Phenytoin
- [ ] B   Isoniazid
- [ ] C   Isotretinoin
- [ ] D   Alcohol
- [ ] E   Sodium valproate

Answers on pages 222–223

21. A 25-year-old man is brought in by ambulance to the Accident and Emergency Department with a Glasgow Coma Scale score of 13/15. It is suspected that he took a drug overdose 12 hours previously but he is unable to remember what he took. For which one of the following is a specific antidote not available?

- ☐ A Ferrous sulphate
- ☐ B Cyanide
- ☐ C Morphine
- ☐ D Amitriptyline
- ☐ E Paracetamol

22. A 70-year-old man has stable, well-controlled atrial fibrillation and has been on digoxin for several years. He presents with nausea, vomiting and confusion. His serum digoxin level is raised. Which one of the following is most likely to exacerbate this problem?

- ☐ A Thyrotoxic heart failure
- ☐ B Left ventricular failure
- ☐ C Captopril
- ☐ D Spironolactone
- ☐ E Warfarin

23. Which one of the following drugs is most likely to cause gynaecomastia?

- ☐ A Diazepam
- ☐ B Methysergide
- ☐ C Metoclopramide
- ☐ D Cimetidine
- ☐ E Clopidogrel

24. **Which one of the following is a known cause of galactorrhoea?**

☐ A Cannabis
☐ B Alcohol
☐ C Digoxin
☐ D Phenothiazine
☐ E Spironolactone

25. **Which one of the following statements about ergotamine is true?**

☐ A It is chemically related to methysergide
☐ B It is a powerful vasodilator
☐ C It is an α-adrenoceptor blocker
☐ D It is safe for use in pregnancy
☐ E It is useful in the prophylaxis of migraine

26. **Which one of the following agents can be used without caution in renal failure?**

☐ A Magnesium trisilicate mixture
☐ B Amphotericin
☐ C Diazepam
☐ D Vancomycin
☐ E Nitrofurantoin

27. **A 67-year-old man with hypertension presents to Casualty with severe central crushing chest pain and breathlessness. On arrival he is hypotensive and tachycardic. His ECG shows an acute anterior myocardial infarct. Following thrombolysis with recombinant tissue plasminogen activator, his blood pressure fails to improve, so he is started on dopamine. Which one of the following effects is a benefit of using dopamine therapy in this situation?**

☐ A Bradycardia
☐ B A rise in diastolic blood pressure
☐ C Arteriolar constriction
☐ D Vasodilatation of the renal vasculature
☐ E Decreased cardiac output

28. Which one of the following drugs characteristically causes an increase in heart rate?

☐ A Glyceryl trinitrate
☐ B Pethidine
☐ C Sotalol
☐ D Amiodarone
☐ E Digoxin

29. A 42-year-old man with rheumatoid arthritis is admitted to hospital with fulminant hepatic failure. A drug-related cause is suspected and all his medication is stopped. His hepatic function begins to recover over the next two weeks. Which one of the following drugs is it safe to recommence without dose adjustment?

☐ A Azathioprine
☐ B Colchicine
☐ C Methotrexate
☐ D Paracetamol
☐ E Tetracycline

30. A 78-year-old man is seen by his general practitioner with a two-day history of haematuria, dysuria and frequency. Dipstick urinalysis is positive for nitrites, leucocytes and blood, and he is treated with a course of oral antibiotics. The problem recurs several times over the next few months and the same antibiotic is used to good effect. One year later he returns to his doctor complaining of burning pain in his hands and feet. Which one of the following antibiotics is he most likely to have received?

☐ A Ciprofloxacin
☐ B Co-amoxiclav
☐ C Nitrofurantoin
☐ D Trimethoprim
☐ E Tetracycline

31. An 80-year-old man complains of a progressive worsening of
     breathlessness over the last six months. On examination, he has
     fine end-expiratory crepitations at his lung bases and a chest X-ray
     shows bilateral basal reticulonodular shadowing. Which one of
     the following drugs is the most likely cause?

     ☐ A   Prednisolone
     ☐ B   Sulfadiazine
     ☐ C   Chloramphenicol
     ☐ D   Colomycin
     ☐ E   Bleomycin

32. A 52-year-old man presents to the Accident and Emergency
     Department with increasing lethargy, breathlessness and episodes
     of epistaxis over the last two weeks. A full blood count reveals the
     following: haemoglobin 5.6 g/dl, WCC 1.6×10^9/l, platelet count
     21×10^9/l. Which one of the following agents is most likely to
     have caused this peripheral blood profile?

     ☐ A   Aspirin
     ☐ B   Gold
     ☐ C   Sulfadiazine
     ☐ D   Sodium valproate
     ☐ E   Paromomycin

33. A 34-year-old woman visits her general practitioner because she
     has had some painful bumps on her legs for a few days. On
     examination, she has multiple, small, tender red lumps on both
     shins. Which one of the following drugs is most likely to have
     caused her lesions?

     ☐ A   Dapsone
     ☐ B   Rifampicin
     ☐ C   Phenobarbital (phenobarbitone)
     ☐ D   Phenytoin
     ☐ E   Oral contraceptive pill

Answers on pages 225–226

34. A 54-year-old woman with rheumatoid arthritis is seen in the Rheumatology Outpatients Clinic. She was diagnosed with the disorder two years ago and has had frequent flare-ups. It was decided on her last visit to commence a disease-modifying agent and gold therapy was started. Unfortunately, she has experienced a number of side effects. Which one of the following is the commonest reported side effect of gold therapy?

- A Mouth ulcers
- B Diarrhoea
- C Peripheral neuropathy
- D Aplastic anaemia
- E Skin pigmentation

35. A 45-year-old man has had epilepsy since he was a teenager. His fits have always been well controlled on oral phenytoin therapy, with, on average, only one seizure every six months. Which of the following is a recognised complication of long-term phenytoin therapy?

- A Ataxia
- B Megaloblastic anaemia
- C Hypercalcaemia
- D Nephrotoxicity
- E Osteoporosis

36. Early on in her pregnancy, a 27-year-old woman develops a painful swollen right leg. A deep vein thrombosis of the right common iliac vein is diagnosed using Doppler ultrasound. As she cannot be given warfarin because of its teratogenicity, she is started on a six-week course of low molecular weight heparin injections. Which one of the following reactions is a recognised side effect of heparin therapy?

- A Muscle pain
- B Osteoporosis
- C Thrombocytosis
- D Hirsutism
- E Hyperkalaemia

37. Which one of the following drugs is safe in patients with glucose-6-phosphate dehydrogenase (G6PD) deficiency?

☐ A Primaquine
☐ B Dapsone
☐ C Ciprofloxacin
☐ D Nitrofurantoin
☐ E Sulphonamides

38. A 29-year-old woman visits her general practitioner. For the last six months she has noticed that her fingers are very painful when her hands are cold. She has also noticed that her fingertips go white, then blue, and then red in cold weather. Which one of the following drugs is most likely to cause these symptoms?

☐ A Clonidine
☐ B Amiodarone
☐ C Isoniazid
☐ D Nitrofurantoin
☐ E Nifedipine

39. A 66-year-old man attends his doctor because of severe pains in his toes. On examination, he has a hot swollen first metatarsophalangeal joint on his right foot. He also has a swelling on the posterior aspect of his right elbow. Which one of the following drugs is most likely to cause this clinical picture?

☐ A High-dose aspirin
☐ B Carbamazepine
☐ C Dapsone
☐ D Pyrazinamide
☐ E Ergotamine

40. **Which one of the following drugs is the safest to continue at the same dose with severe renal impairment?**

- ☐ A Digoxin
- ☐ B Ranitidine
- ☐ C Metronidazole
- ☐ D Gentamicin
- ☐ E Non-steroidal anti-inflammatory drugs (NSAIDs)

41. **Which one of the following statements is most true regarding poisoning?**

- ☐ A Ethylene glycol leads to a metabolic alkalosis
- ☐ B Aminophylline overdose leads to hyperkalaemia
- ☐ C N-acetylcysteine improves mortality in hepatic encephalopathy
- ☐ D Charcoal haemoperfusion increases elimination of phenobarbital (phenobarbitone)
- ☐ E Salicylate overdose is managed with a single dose of activated charcoal

42. **Breakthrough bleeding or pregnancy may occur in a woman who is taking both the combined oral contraceptive pill and which one of the following drugs?**

- ☐ A Cimetidine
- ☐ B Sodium valproate
- ☐ C Ciprofloxacin
- ☐ D Carbamazepine
- ☐ E Indometacin

43. **Which one of the following pairings of cytotoxic drug and adverse effect is correct?**

- ☐ A Busulfan – pulmonary oedema
- ☐ B Cyclophosphamide – haemorrhagic cystitis
- ☐ C Methotrexate – cardiomyopathy
- ☐ D Doxorubicin – peripheral neuropathy
- ☐ E Vincristine – encephalopathy

44. **Which one of the following statements about sodium valproate is most true?**

☐ A   It is a useful mood stabiliser
☐ B   It can cause permanent hair loss
☐ C   It can cause rapid weight loss
☐ D   It can cause fatal nephrotoxicity
☐ E   It induces liver enzymes

45. **Which one of the following is a recognised side effect of thiazides?**

☐ A   Pancreatitis
☐ B   Anaemia
☐ C   Hyperchloraemia
☐ D   Hypermagnesaemia
☐ E   Urinary incontinence

46. **A 52-year-old man with known hypertrophic cardiomyopathy presents to his general practitioner with a history of rapid palpitations over the past week. An ECG confirms a rhythm disturbance. His doctor commences him on a medication and books him in for a repeat ECG two weeks later. This reveals a worsening of his left ventricular outflow tract obstruction. In keeping with this, he now reports that he has had several syncopal episodes. Which one of the following medications has he probably been prescribed?**

☐ A   Amiodarone
☐ B   Digoxin
☐ C   Verapamil
☐ D   Sotalol
☐ E   Atenolol

47. A 66-year-old man with end-stage renal failure, who is on haemodialysis, is admitted with a five-hour history of chest pain. He has a past history of hypertension and type 1 diabetes mellitus. An ECG shows inferior ST-segment depression and new-onset atrial fibrillation. The troponin-I level is also raised. Which one of the following drugs is contraindicated in this situation?

☐ A Aspirin
☐ B Clopidogrel
☐ C Unfractionated heparin
☐ D Low molecular weight heparin
☐ E Warfarin

48. A 56-year-old man with known ischaemic heart disease presents to his general practitioner with a one-year history of erectile dysfunction. He suffers from grade II angina and occasionally uses his glyceryl trinitrate (GTN) spray. He is also currently on a course of erythromycin for a chest infection. He is keen to know if he can be prescribed Viagra®. Which one of the following is true regarding sildenafil?

☐ A It is contraindicated in ischaemic heart disease
☐ B Its effect is increased when it is given with erythromycin
☐ C Its action is mediated via reduction of nitric oxide (NO) levels
☐ D It is used with nitrates to enhance its effect in resistant cases
☐ E A rare but serious side effect is primary pulmonary hypertension

49. A 24-year-old man is brought to the Accident and Emergency Department with a Glasgow Coma Scale score of 10/15 after being found collapsed outside a nightclub. His core temperature is 41 °C, his blood pressure is 210/110 mmHg, and he has a grand mal seizure on arrival. Active cooling is commenced and he is given intravenous lorazepam. Initial electrolytes reveal the following: Na$^+$ 119 mmol/l, K$^+$ 6.2 mmol/l, urea 14 mmol/l, creatinine 230 μmol/l, creatine kinase 4568 U/l. Which one of the following substances is he most likely to have taken?

- [ ] A γ-Hydroxybutyrate (GHB)
- [ ] B Lysergic acid diethylamide (LSD)
- [ ] C Methylenedioxymethamfetamine (MDMA)
- [ ] D Cocaine
- [ ] E Diamorphine

50. A 26-year-old man is admitted to hospital with a four-day history of a widespread blistering rash, oral ulcers, general malaise and arthralgia. His blood tests reveal: WCC 15.2 × 10^9/l (eosinophils 8.2 × 10^9/l, neutrophils 4.4 × 10^9/l), bilirubin 67 μmol/l, ALT 457 U/l, ALP 100 U/l, AST 356 U/l. He is HIV-positive and was commenced on antiretroviral therapy one week previously. Which one of the following drugs is most likely to have caused the above reaction?

- [ ] A Zidovudine
- [ ] B Lamuvidine
- [ ] C Efavirenz
- [ ] D Nevirapine
- [ ] E Abacavir

PHARMACOLOGY

Answers

1. C: Lithium

Lithium is excreted in breast milk and may cause involuntary movements and tremor in the neonate. Insulin-dependent diabetic mothers are encouraged to breastfeed their infants.

2. B: They accumulate in tissues as treatment progresses

Aminoglycosides are cleared almost completely by the kidneys, but are nephrotoxic in high doses. They also accumulate in tissues, even when serum levels are within normal limits. They are inactive against streptococcal groups A, B, C and G and *Streptococcus pneumoniae*. Toxicity may occur up to one week after treatment has finished. Adverse effects are unlikely if the peak serum concentration of gentamicin is less than 10 μg/ml and the trough is less than 2 μg/ml. The risk of ototoxicty increases with the concomitant use of loop diuretics. An inherited tendency to aminoglycoside ototoxicity is transmitted on mitochondrial DNA.

3. D: Enalapril

Methyldopa is safe to treat hypertension in pregnancy. Hydralazine is safe to use in the third trimester, although not recommended before this. Most β-blockers can cause intrauterine growth retardation, but labetolol is licensed for use in pregnancy. Calcium-channel blockers, such as amlodipine and nifedipine are considered safe, although diltiazem has been shown to be teratogenic in animals. All angiotension-converting enzyme (ACE) inhibitors are contraindicated as they can cause problems with renal development and oligohydramnios.

4. **D: Meropenem**

    Erythromycin and rifampicin are cleared by the liver. Metronidazole is excreted via the liver and gastrointestinal tract. There is significant renal excretion of furosemide (frusemide), and the dose of furosemide should be increased in renal failure. Meropenem is excreted by the kidney and should be dose-adjusted.

5. **D: Magnesium trisilicate**

    Tricyclic antidepressants and disopyramide have anticholinergic properties which may cause constipation. Antacids containing calcium carbonate or aluminium hydroxide cause constipation, but magnesium salts cause diarrhoea. Colestyramine may be used to treat diarrhoea caused by bile salt malabsorption.

6. **E: Lithium**

    Carbamazepine, desmopressin (an arginine vasopressin analogue) and cyclophosphamide cause hyponatraemia through the stimulation of antidiuretic hormone (ADH) secretion. Lithium causes hypernatraemia as a result of nephrogenic diabetes insipidus.

7. **C: Colestyramine**

    Enalapril is metabolised to the active compound, enalaprilat. Isosorbide dinitrate is metabolised to the mononitrate which, if taken orally, provides more predictable blood levels. Colestyramine is a resin, which is not absorbed. The relatively high doses of ethinylestradiol to which the liver is exposed in order to deliver adequate concentrations may be responsible for some of the adverse effects of oestrogen therapy.

8. **B: Co-trimoxazole**

Lithium decreases the hypoglycaemic effect of sulphonylureas. Co-trimoxazole and other sulphonamides displace protein-bound sulphonylureas and increase the hypoglycaemic effect. Rifampicin and phenytoin are hepatic enzyme inducers and so reduce the hypoglycaemic effect. Thiazide diuretics may cause a deterioration in glucose tolerance.

9. **C: Colestyramine**

Calcium-channel blockers do not have an adverse effect on serum lipid profiles. Colestyramine causes increased hepatic synthesis and secretion of triglycerides.

10. **B: It is contraindicated in severe neutropenia**

Zidovudine is a nucleoside reverse transcriptase inhibitor, which is a structural analogue of thymidine, with an oral bioavailability of 65%. The drug has a serum half-life of one hour but the half-life of the active intracellular triphosphate moiety is three hours. It is a known cause of myelosuppression and is usually given twice a day.

11. **A: Chlorpromazine**

Drugs which precipitate attacks of acute intermittent porphyria include hepatic enzyme inducers (eg rifampicin, phenytoin, sulphonamides, sulphonylureas), the oral contraceptive pill, ACE inhibitors, calcium-channel blockers and furosemide (frusemide). Drugs which are safe to use include paracetamol, aspirin, codeine, morphine, penicillin, β-blockers and metformin.

12. **B: Chlorpropramide**

Aspirin potentiates the effects of oral hypoglycaemics, warfarin, non-steroidal anti-inflammatory drugs (NSAIDs), steroids and alcohol.

13. E: Erythromycin

Aminoglycosides and tetracyclines are directly nephrotoxic, and may cause an acute tubular necrosis. An acute interstitial nephritis may be caused by penicillins, tetracyclines, sulphonamides, rifampicin and streptomycin.

14. B: Co-trimoxazole

Monoamine-oxidase inhibitors (MAOIs) cause an accumulation of amine neurotransmitters, and therefore the use of sympathomimetic amines should be avoided. These include tricyclic antidepressants, L-dopa, barbiturates, amphetamines and pethidine. Any food containing tyrosine (eg red wine, soft cheese, Bovril®) should be avoided as MAOIs can potentiate the pressor effect of tyrosine. The interaction of these agents with MAOIs can lead to a hypertensive crisis, with CNS excitation and sometimes hyperpyrexia, as well as prolongation of the action of the interacting drugs.

15. A: Doxycycline

Other drugs which can cause a photosensitivity reaction include amiodarone, oestrogens and progesterones, sulphonamides, griseofulvin, phenothiazines, chlordiazepoxide and ACE inhibitors. Although benzodiazepines have been known to cause photosensitivity, the incidence with tetracyclines is much higher.

16. C: Digoxin and erythromycin

Rifampicin is a hepatic enzyme inducer and reduces the action of the oral contraceptive pill. Other hepatic enzyme inducers include phenytoin, carbamazepine, phenobarbital (phenobarbitone), isoniazid, chloramphenicol and griseofulvin. Chloral hydrate may increase the anticoagulant effect of warfarin. Monoamine-oxidase inhibitors increase the effect of L-dopa. Beta-blockers enhance digoxin toxicity.

PHARMACOLOGY – **ANSWERS**

17. C: Halothane

Intrahepatic cholestatic jaundice and hepatitis may be caused by tricyclic antidepressants, phenothiazines, NSAIDs, rifampicin, erythromycin, sulphonamides and sulphonylureas. Norethandrolone and the oral contraceptive pill cause cholestasis alone. Carbon tetrachloride is a direct hepatotoxin. Repeated administration of halothane, and exposure to isoniazid, pyrazinamide, rifampicin, monoamine-oxidase inhibitors, methyldopa and anticonvulsants, may cause an acute hepatitis two to three weeks after exposure.

18. B: Toxicity is associated with a macrocytic anaemia

Phenytoin has a narrow therapeutic range and the relationship between dose and plasma concentration is non-linear. Phenytoin displaces iodine from its protein-binding sites. The long-term side effects of phenytoin include folate deficiency and megaloblastic anaemia. Phenytoin toxicity causes a cerebellar syndrome.

19. E: Amiodarone

Therapeutic drug level monitoring is required for drugs which have a narrow therapeutic range (eg lithium) or for drugs with dose-dependent pharmacokinetics (eg phenytoin). Drug level monitoring is available for:

1. Antiarrhythmics – procainamide and quinidine
2. Antibiotics – aminoglycosides
3. Anticonvulsants – phenobarbital (phenobarbitone), phenytoin and carbamazepine
4. Others – digoxin, aminophylline, lithium.

20. B: Isoniazid

Phenytoin causes cleft palate, microcephaly and mental retardation, and screening is advised. Retinoids may cause hydrocephalus and neural tube defects. Alcohol in high concentrations causes the fetal alcohol syndrome. Sodium valproate may cause neural tube defects.

21. D: Amitriptyline

The antidote for iron poisoning is desferrioxamine; for paracetamol it is N-acetylcysteine or methionine; for morphine or other opiates it is naloxone, an oral opiate antagonist; and for cyanide it is sodium thiosulphate or cobalt edetate.

22. B: Left ventricular failure

Digoxin toxicity is depends on the plasma concentration of the drug and on the myocardial sensitivity to it (often increased in heart failure). Toxicity is more likely in the presence of hypokalaemia, so diuretic therapy given with digoxin should either be potassium-sparing or given with potassium supplements. Digoxin toxicity is exacerbated by hypercalcaemia, verapamil, β-blockers, amiodarone and quinidine.

23. D: Cimetidine

Other drugs associated with gynaecomastia include tricyclic antidepressants, cytotoxic agents, phenothiazines, spironolactone, diethylstilbestrol (stilboestrol), digoxin and methyldopa. Methysergide may cause retroperitoneal fibrosis.

24. D: Phenothiazine

Other drugs associated with galactorrhoea include cimetidine, metoclopramide, L-dopa, oestrogens and benzodiazepines. Cannabis, alcohol, digoxin and spironolactone are all known causes of gynaecomastia.

25. A: It is chemically related to methysergide

Ergotamine is a powerful α-adrenoreceptor blocker. Side effects include abdominal pain and vomiting. Repeated administration of high doses may cause ergotism with gangrene and confusion. It is licensed for use in the treatment of migraine in patients who do not have any contraindications. It causes post-partum contraction of the uterus. Pleural and peritoneal fibrosis may occur, as with methysergide.

26. **C: Diazepam**

    The following drugs should be avoided in renal failure:

    - antimicrobial drugs (amphotericin B, tetracyclines, nitrofurantoin)
    - aspirin and NSAIDs
    - lithium
    - narcotic analgesics
    - potassium-sparing diuretics.

    The following drugs should have their dose reduced when used in renal failure:

    - antimicrobials (aminoglycosides, vancomycin, sulphonamides, cephalosporins, penicillin, metronidazole)
    - cardiac drugs (digoxin, methyldopa, procainamide, disopyramide)
    - insulin
    - chlorpropramide
    - H_2-antagonists.

27. **D: Vasodilatation of the renal vasculature**

    Dopamine is an agonist at β_1 receptors in cardiac muscle. It is a positive inotrope, increasing myocardial contractility with little effect on rate, and is therefore used in cardiogenic shock. The dose of dopamine used is very important. Standard doses of <5 micrograms/kg/minute induce vasodilatation and increase renal perfusion, whereas higher doses may lead to vasoconstriction and heart failure.

28. **A: Glyceryl trinitrate**

    Glyceryl trinitrate is a potent coronary vasodilator, but its main mode of action is reduction of venous return, which reduces left ventricular work. Side effects include throbbing headaches, flushing, postural hypotension and tachycardia.

29. B: Colchicine

Azathioprine, methotrexate, paracetamol and tetracycline are all directly hepatotoxic. Other directly hepatotoxic agents include carbon tetrachloride, 6-mercaptopurine and aflatoxin.

30. C: Nitrofurantoin

Other agents which cause a peripheral neuropathy include metronidazole, chloramphenicol, streptomycin, ethambutol, sulphonylureas, phenelzine and tricyclic antidepressants.

31. E: Bleomycin

Other drugs which cause pulmonary fibrosis include amiodarone, azathioprine, busulfan, chlorambucil, methotrexate, methysergide, nitrofurantoin, sulfasalazine, and prolonged high-dose oxygen.

32. B: Gold

Drugs which may cause aplastic anaemia include:

- anti-arrhythmics – quinidine, procainamide
- antibiotics – sulphonamides, methicillin, ampicillin, chloramphenicol, co-trimoxazole
- anticonvulsants – phenytoin, carbamazepine
- antimalarials – chloroquine, pyrimethamine
- antirheumatic agents – penicillamine, gold salts
- antithyroid agents – carbimazole
- cytotoxic agents
- diuretics – thiazides, furosemide (frusemide)
- oral hypoglycaemics – sulphonylureas
- phenothiazines
- tricyclic antidepressants.

33. E: Oral contraceptive pill

Other drugs which may cause erythema nodosum include sulphonamides, salicylates, penicillins, phenylbutazone, sulphonylureas and gold salts. Dapsone has also been reported to cause erythema nodosum, but to a far lesser degree than the oral contraceptive pill.

34. B: Diarrhoea

The most common side effect of oral gold therapy is diarrhoea, which may occur with or without abdominal pain. Severe adverse reactions occur in up to 5% of patients and include aplastic anaemia, proteinuria, pulmonary fibrosis, alopecia, mouth ulcers, peripheral neuritis and cholestatic jaundice.

35. B: Megaloblastic anaemia

Other long-term effects of phenytoin therapy include gingival hyperplasia, hypocalcaemia, hypersensitivity reactions, rashes, SLE syndrome and lymphadenopathy. Ataxia is more often seen with toxic serum levels of phenytoin rather than as a consequence of long-term therapy.

36. B: Osteoporosis

Hypersensitivity reactions to heparin therapy include rhinitis, urticaria, angio-oedema and anaphylaxis. Thrombocytopenia may occur. With long-term treatment, osteoporosis and alopecia are recognised effects.

37. C: Ciprofloxacin

'Oxidant' drugs which should be avoided in patients with G6PD deficiency include:

* analgesics – aspirin, phenacetin
* antimicrobials – chloramphenicol, sulphonamides, nitrofurantoin, dapsone, co-trimoxazole
* antimalarials – chloroquine, primaquine, quinine
* quinidine
* probenecid.

38. A: Clonidine

Clonidine causes Raynaud's phenomenon. Other side effects include sedation, depression, fluid retention, dry mouth, impotence and bradycardia. Sudden withdrawal may cause a hypertensive crisis. Beta-blockers and ergotamine are also known causes of the phenomenon. Stopping smoking can greatly ease the severity of Raynaud's. Nifedipine is used in its treatment.

39. D: Pyrazinamide

Drugs which cause hyperuricaemia include loop and thiazide diuretics, alcohol, ethambutol, pyrazinamide and cytotoxic agents. Low-dose aspirin usage is also associated, but high-dose aspirin may be used to treat the condition.

40. C: Metronidazole

See answer to Question 26.

41. D: Charcoal haemoperfusion increases elimination of phenobarbital (phenobarbitone)

Profound hypokalaemia may develop rapidly after overdosage with theophylline and related drugs. Forced alkaline diuresis and charcoal haemoperfusion are the treatment options for the small minority of patients with very severe barbiturate poisoning who fail to improve despite supportive care. Acetylcysteine may protect the liver if given within 10–12 hours of ingestion of paracetamol, but there is no conclusive evidence for its usefulness in hepatic disease due to other causes. Ethylene glycol causes a metabolic acidosis. Salicylate poisoning is one of few scenarios in which repeated doses of activated charcoal may be beneficial.

42. D: Carbamazepine

Carbamazepine is a hepatic enzyme inducer, and may decrease the effectiveness of the oral contraceptive. Other drugs with a similar effect include phenytoin, rifampicin, isoniazid and griseofulvin. Cimetidine, ciprofloxacin and sodium valproate are hepatic enzyme inhibitors.

43. **B: Cyclophosphamide – haemorrhagic cystitis**

Other characteristic side effects of these cytotoxic drugs include:

- bulsulphan – pulmonary fibrosis, skin pigmentation, aplastic anaemia
- cyclophosphamide – haemorrhagic cystitis, skin pigmentation
- doxorubicin – cardiomyopathy
- methotrexate – hepatotoxicity, pneumonitis, mucositis, encephalopathy
- vincristine – joint pain, paralytic ileus, peripheral neuropathy, hyponatraemia.

44. **A: It is a useful mood stabiliser**

The plasma concentration of sodium valproate is not a useful index of efficacy, so routine monitoring is unhelpful. Sodium valproate is a hepatic enzyme inhibitor. Other side effects include ataxia, tremor, oedema, thrombocytopenia, amenorrhoea, leucopenia, gynaecomastia and transient hair loss. It has been known to cause rapid weight gain and rarely results in fatal hepatotoxicity. It is increasingly being used in bipolar affective disorder as a mood stabiliser.

45. **C: Hyperchloraemia**

Other potential side effects of thiazides include hypochloraemia, hypokalaemia, hypomagnesaemia, hyperglycaemia, hyperuricaemia, acute urinary retention, rashes, agranulocytosis, thrombocytopenia and inhibition of calcium excretion.

46. B: Digoxin

At a cellular level digoxin blocks the exchange of intracellular Na^+ for extracellular K^+ by inhibiting the Na^+/K^+ ATPase in the cell membrane. This increases intracellular Na^+ and encourages its exchange for Ca^{2+}, raising intracellular Ca^{2+} and thus causing a weak positive inotropic effect. This in turn leads to aggravation of the left ventricular outflow tract obstruction in hypertrophic obstructive cardiomyopathy (HOCM). Both β-blockers and calcium-channel antagonists are used to relieve the obstruction pharmacologically. Evidence regarding the benefit of amiodarone is controversial, but may it be helpful in elderly patients with HOCM and atrial fibrillation or non-sustained ventricular tachycardia.

47. D: Low molecular weight heparin

The low molecular weight heparins (LMWH) are purified derivatives that have more consistent activity, require less monitoring, and have a longer duration of action than unfractionated heparin. They are now widely used in place of unfractionated heparin in the treatment of acute coronary syndrome and in thromboembolic disease. They are contraindicated in severe renal impairment, however, due to the risk of accumulation. Factor Xa levels would need to be monitored in order to use LMWH safely in renal impairment, which is not practical in most UK hospitals.

48. B: Its effect is increased when it is given with erythromycin

Erectile response is mediated by the release of nitric oxide (NO) from nerves supplying vessels in the corpora cavernosa. This increases intracellular cGMP levels, which in turn causes vasodilatation. This effect is terminated by phosphodiesterase type 5 enzyme, which is inhibited selectively by sildenafil, thus enhancing the vasodilatory effects of NO. Inhibitors of the CYP3A4 enzyme system, such as erythromycin, ketoconazole, protease inhibitors and cimetidine, all increase blood levels of sildenafil. Concurrent administration with nitrates is contraindicated due to the risk of profound, fatal hypotension. It is currently indicated, but unlicensed, in primary pulmonary hypertension.

49. C: Methylenedioxymethamfetamine (MDMA)

Ecstacy (methylenedioxymethamfetamine, MDMA) is a drug used widely for recreational purposes and acts mainly by increasing 5-HT (serotonin) release into synaptic clefts in the central nervous system. It therefore also depletes intracellular stores of serotonin. It can cause a syndrome of hyperpyrexia, hypertension, hyponatraemia (due either to excess sodium loss through sweating or to syndrome of inappopriate ADH secretion, SIADH), rhabdomyolysis (and acute renal failure), and seizures. Disseminated intravascular coagulation is also seen. Management is supportive, with active cooling (tepid sponging, paracetamol), benzodiazepines for seizures and calcium-channel antagonists for hypertension. Intravenous dantrolene (a non-specific skeletal muscle relaxant) is also used to good effect, as in malignant hyperthermia due to anaesthetic agents and in neuroleptic malignant syndrome.

50. D: Nevirapine

Nevirapine is a non-nucleoside reverse transcriptase inhibitor, which is widely used in first-line combination therapy in treatment-naïve patients. It can result in a severe rash, eosinophilia and hepatitis syndrome. It should be permanently discontinued and the patient treated supportively. It can sometimes cause an extremely severe Stevens–Johnson syndrome. Abacavir, a nucleoside reverse transcriptase inhibitor, can also result in hypersensitivity reactions, characterised by a rash, anaphylaxis, abdominal pain and diarrhoea. These symptoms typically get worse with each extra dose taken. Efavirenz typically causes psychiatric disturbance and vivid dreams.

INDEX

Locators are given as chapter number.question number

ABO blood groups   6.11
ACE inhibitors   9.3
acid phosphatase   7.7
acid–base balance   6.2–3, 6.21–2
acidosis   6.3, 7.31
Acinetobacter baumanii   3.37
acute phase response   4.18, 7.37
adrenalectomy   7.25
adrenergic neurones   6.37
AIDS *see* HIV
airway obstruction   6.10
alcohol abuse   7.4
alkaline phosphatase   7.28
alkalosis   6.2, 6.21
allergy *see* hypersensitivity
α-fetoprotein   1.17
$α_1$-antitrypsin deficiency   1.18
altitude sickness   6.53
aminoglycosides   2.16, 9.2
amniotic fluid AFP   1.17
anaemia
    drug-induced   9.32
    erythropoietin   6.12
    pernicious   7.12
aneuploidy   1.8, 1.10–13
angiotensin   6.28
antibiotics
    aminoglycosides   2.16, 9.2
    mode of action   2.23
    penicillins   3.4
    resistance   3.19, 3.25, 3.38

side-effects   9.13, 9.30
antibodies *see* autoantibodies;
    immunoglobulins
antidiuretic hormone (ADH)   6.18
anti-emetics   6.46
antigens
    antigenic variation   4.25
    presentation to T cells   4.29–30
antimitochondrial antibodies   4.28
antinuclear antibodies   4.11
antioxidants   2.19
antiphospholipid antibody (APA)
    syndrome   4.24
antisense technology   2.20
antiviral drugs   3.34, 9.10, 9.50
aorta, abdominal   5.6
apoptosis   2.7
appetite suppressants   6.51
arm *see* upper limb
aspirin   9.12
asthma   4.17
atropine   5.29
autoantibodies
    ANA   4.11
    antimitochondrial   4.28
    APA   4.24
    c-ANCA   4.19
    rashes caused by   4.31
autonomic nervous system
    adrenergic   6.37
    parasympathetic   6.38

autonomic nervous system (*cont.*)
  sympathetic 6.17, 6.38

BCG vaccination 4.15
Bell's palsy 5.14
β-lactam antibiotics 3.19, 3.25
bilirubin 6.19
blood gases
  acid–base balance 6.2–3,
    6.21–2
  binding to haemoglobin 6.27,
    6.47, 7.27
  carbon dioxide 6.21
  cerebral blood flow 6.35
  ventilation control 6.7
blood groups 6.11
blood pressure
  control 6.13, 6.31, 6.50
  hypertension 2.1, 9.3
  hypotension 6.4, 6.28
blood–brain barrier 6.32
brachial plexus 5.21
brain
  blood flow 6.35
  blood–brain barrier 6.32
  CSF 6.33, 7.3
  damage 5.24, 5.31–2
  intracranial pressure 6.41
  see also cranial nerves
breastfeeding 9.1
breathing *see* ventilation
bronchus 5.3
Bruton's congenital
    agammaglobulinaemia 4.22
busulphan 9.43

C-reactive protein (CRP) 7.37
calcium
  hypercalcaemia 7.16, 7.22
  hypercalciuria 7.23
carbon dioxide 6.21
carcinogenesis
  familial colon cancer 1.21
  proto-oncogenes 2.4
  tumour suppressor genes 1.15, 2.5,
    2.9
cardiogenic shock 5.30, 9.27
cardiovascular system *see* heart

case–control (retrospective) studies
    8.6, 8.16–17
causality 8.16
CD antigens/cells 4.5, 4.27, 4.33,
    4.36
cell death (apoptosis) 2.7
cell senescence 2.21
cell signalling
  transduction 2.6, 2.12
  see also cytokines
cerebrospinal fluid (CSF)
  low globulin:albumin ratio 7.3
  normal 6.33
cerebrovascular accident 5.24, 5.32
Charcot–Marie–Tooth disease 1.14
chemoreceptor trigger zone (CTZ)
    6.46
chi-squared tests 8.4
chloride 7.31
cholera 2.6
cholesterol 7.35
cholinergic neurones 6.37
chromosome abnormalities 1.8,
    1.10–13
circulatory system, peripheral 6.13,
    6.50
Clinitest® reaction 7.5
clonidine 9.38
coagulation 4.24, 6.15–16
cohort (prospective) studies 8.6, 8.16
colestyramine 9.7, 9.9
colon cancer, familial 1.21
complement 4.8
confidence intervals 8.8
congenital infections 3.2, 3.10, 3.12
conjugation, bacterial 3.30
connective tissue diseases 4.11, 4.19
constipation 9.5
contraception *see* oral contraceptives
correlation coefficients 8.5, 8.12
corticospinal pathway 5.25
corticosteroids 7.24
cortisol 6.9
Coxiella burnetii 3.36
cranial nerves 5.14, 5.23, 5.26
creatinine 6.23
Creutzfeldt–Jakob disease (CJD) 3.14
cri-du-chat syndrome 1.8

CRP (C-reactive protein) 7.37
Cryptosporidium parvum 3.28
cyclooxygenases (COX) 7.36
cyclophosphamide 9.43
cystic fibrosis 1.6, 2.22
cystinuria 1.9
cytokines
 IL-1 2.3
 interferons 2.15, 3.34, 4.23,
  4.26
 production by T cells 4.27
 TGF-β 2.18
 TNF 2.8, 4.14
cytoplasmic-staining antineutrophil
  cytoplasmic antibodies
  (c-ANCA) 4.19
cytotoxic drugs 9.43

dermatitis herpetiformis 4.31
diabetes
 hypoglycaemia 6.26, 9.8
 inheritance 1.22
 insulin metabolism 7.8
diarrhoea
 drug-related 9.5
 E. coli 3.13, 3.27
digoxin 9.16, 9.22, 9.46
diphtheria 3.16
distribution, statistical 8.1–3, 8.8–9,
  8.11
DNA
 antisense technology 2.20
 bacterial transfer 3.30
 PCR 2.10
 structure 1.7
 trinucleotide repeats 2.13
dobutamine 5.30
dopamine 9.27
Down's syndrome 1.12
doxorubicin 9.43
dystrophin 2.19

Ebola virus disease 3.5, 3.33
Ecstasy (MDMA) 9.49
electrocardiograms (ECGs) 6.40,
  6.48
electrolyte balance
 Fanconi syndrome 7.38

physiology 6.24, 6.42
see also individual electrolytes
electromyograms (EMGs) 6.34
emphysema 1.18, 6.52
encephalitis 7.3
endocarditis 3.26, 3.36
endothelin 2.1
Enterococcus faecalis 3.26
epidemiological studies 8.6, 8.13,
  8.16–17, 8.19
ergotamine 9.25
erythema infectiosum 3.23
erythema nodosum 9.33
erythropoietin 6.12
Escherichia coli 3.13, 3.27
exotoxins 3.16

facial nerve 5.14
Fanconi syndrome 7.38
fat metabolism 6.43, 7.9
femoral nerve 5.4
flaviviruses 3.5
flow cytometry 4.36
foot 5.13, 5.22

G proteins 2.6
galactorrhoea 9.24
gas transfer factor 6.8
gastrin 6.39
Gaucher's disease 7.7
gene therapy 2.22
genome structure 1.19
gentamicin 2.16, 9.2
glomerular filtration rate (GFR) 6.23,
  6.25
glucocorticoids 7.24
glucose
 gluconeogenesis 7.9, 7.20, 7.25
 glycosuria 7.5
 hypoglycaemia 6.26, 7.14, 7.18,
  7.25, 9.8
glucose-6-phosphate dehydrogenase
  deficiency
 drugs to avoid 9.37
 inheritance 1.3
glyceryl trinitrate 9.28
glycogen storage disorders 7.1
gold therapy 9.34

gout 7.32, 9.39
Guillain–Barré syndrome 6.49
gynaecomastia 9.23

haem, synthesis 7.26
haematuria 7.10
haemoglobin
    Hb S 1.20
    physiology 6.27, 6.47, 7.27
haemophilia 1.4
Haemophilus influenzae 3.3
haemorrhage
    pulmonary 6.56
    shock 6.4
hantaviruses 3.35
heart
    arrhythmias 6.1, 7.34
    drugs affecting 5.29–30, 9.16,
        9.22, 9.27–8, 9.46
    failure 6.5, 6.55
    HOCM 1.16, 6.54, 9.46
    physiology 6.40, 6.48
heat shock proteins 2.19
Helicobacter pylori 3.24
hemianopia 5.23
heparin 9.36, 9.47
hepatitis
    B 3.6, 3.31
    C 3.21
    drug-induced 9.17
high-density lipoprotein cholesterol
    7.35
HIV
    antiretroviral therapy 9.10, 9.50
    diagnosis 4.6
    lymphocytes 4.5
    staging 3.7, 3.39, 4.36
    vaccine use 3.20
    viricides 3.32
homocystinuria 7.13
HTLV-1/3 3.5
human chorionic gonadotrophin
    (HCG) 6.30
human leucocyte antigens (HLA) 1.5
hydrogen ions 6.22
hypersensitivity
    type IV (delayed) 4.13
    type V 4.4

typology 4.3
hypertension
    drug therapy 9.3
    endothelin 2.1
hyperthermia, malignant 1.1
hypertrophic obstructive
    cardiomyopathy (HOCM)
    inheritance 1.16
    outflow tract obstruction 6.54
    treatment 9.46
hyperuricaemia 7.32, 9.39
hypogammaglobulinaemia 4.10
hypoglycaemia 6.26, 7.14, 7.18,
    7.25, 9.8
hypotension 6.4, 6.28

ileum, resection 6.6
immune system
    autoimmune diseases 4.11, 4.19,
        4.24, 4.28, 4.31
    immune complex diseases 4.12
    immunodeficiency diseases 4.22,
        4.34
    innate/adaptive responses 4.18,
        4.32, 7.37
immunoglobulins
    IgA 4.16, 4.20
    IgE 4.9
    IgG 4.9–10, 4.22
    IgM 4.7, 4.21
    monoclonal 2.11
    treatment with 2.11, 4.20
incidence 8.19
inferior vena cava (IVC) 5.20
inheritance
    dominant 1.1, 1.16
    mitochondrial DNA 2.16
    multifactorial disorders 1.21–2
    recessive 1.2, 1.6, 1.9,
        1.18
    X-linked 1.3–4
insulin 6.29, 7.8
integrins 2.19
interactions between drugs 9.8, 9.12,
    9.14, 9.16, 9.42
interferons 2.15, 3.34, 4.23, 4.26
interleukin-1 (IL-1) 2.3
ion channels 7.34

iron 7.6, 7.19
ivermectin 3.29

jugular vein 5.18

ketoacidosis 7.8
kidney
    drug therapy in patients with renal
        failure 9.4, 9.26, 9.40, 9.47
    drugs causing renal failure 9.13
    Fanconi syndrome 7.38
    physiology 6.23–5
    proteinuria 7.21
    renal tubular acidosis 7.23, 7.31
    transplantation 4.1
Klinefelter's syndrome 1.11

Lassa fever 3.5
lead poisoning 7.11
leg see lower limb
Legionella pneumophila 3.8
leptin 6.51
leukotrienes 4.17
Li–Fraumeni syndrome 2.9
linezolid 3.38
lipids 6.43, 7.9, 7.35, 9.9
Listeria monocytogenes 3.2
lithium 9.1, 9.6
liver
    antimitochondrial antibodies 4.28
    drug metabolism 9.7, 9.16, 9.42
    drug-induced failure 9.17, 9.29
lower limb
    muscles 5.22
    nerves 5.2, 5.4, 5.9–10, 5.13, 5.15
lung
    drug-induced fibrosis 9.31
    function tests 6.8, 6.49, 6.52
    haemorrhage 6.56
    infections 3.3, 3.8, 3.17
luteinising hormone
    releasing-hormone (LHRH) 6.45
lymphatic system 5.7
lymphocytes see T cells

magnesium 7.29
major histocompatibility complex
    (MHC) 4.2, 4.29

malaria
    resistance 1.20
    treatment 3.40
mean 8.1–3, 8.9
median (statistics) 8.9
median nerve 5.8
medullary syndrome 5.32
memory 5.31
meningitis 3.1, 3.39
meropenem 9.4
methotrexate 9.43
methylenedioxymethamfetamine
    (MDMA, Ecstasy) 9.49
mitochondrial DNA 2.16
mode 8.1
monoamine-oxidase inhibitors
    (MAOIs) 9.14
monoclonal antibodies 2.11
motor neurone lesions 5.25
mountain sickness 6.53
MRSA (methicillin-resistant
    S. aureus) 3.38
multiple prescribing 9.8, 9.12, 9.14,
    9.16, 9.42
muscles
    controlling the foot 5.22
    electromyograms 6.34
    innervation 5.9
Mycobacterium tuberculosis 3.17
myocardial infarction, drugs 9.27,
    9.47

Neisseria meningitidis 3.1, 3.4
nematodes 3.29
nephrotic syndrome 7.21
neural tube defects 1.17
neuropathy, drug-induced 9.30
nevirapine 9.50
nitric oxide (NO) 2.2, 9.48
non-parametric tests 8.11
non-steroidal anti-inflammatory drugs
    (NSAIDs) 6.55, 9.12
nosocomial infections 3.19, 3.37
null hypothesis 8.14
number needed to treat 8.18

oesophagus 5.16
oncogenes, proto-oncogenes 2.4

opportunistic infections 3.37
optic neurology 5.23
oral contraceptives 9.33, 9.42
osteomyelitis 3.9
ototoxicity 2.16
overdose 9.21, 9.41, 9.49
oxygen
   binding to haemoglobin 6.27,
     6.47, 7.27
   hypoxia 6.53

p53 gene (*TP53*) 1.15, 2.5, 2.9
pain 6.44
pancytopenia 6.6
paraparesis 1.14
parasitic infections 3.29, 7.12
parasympathetic nervous system
   6.38
parvovirus B19 3.23
pemphigoid 4.31
pemphigus 4.31
penetrance, genetic 1.16
penicillins 3.4, 3.19, 3.25
perfusion scans 6.8
peroneal nerve 5.13
pH 6.21–2
phenylketonuria 7.2
phenytoin 9.18, 9.35
phosphate 7.33
photosensitivity, drug-induced 9.15
Plasmodium falciparum 1.20
Plasmodium vivax 3.40
platelets 6.16
pneumonia 3.3, 3.8
poisoning 9.21, 9.41
   lead 7.11
polymerase chain reaction (PCR)
   2.10
porphyria
   acute intermittent 7.15, 7.17, 7.26,
     9.11
   congenital 7.10
portal system 5.12
positive predictive value 8.10
potassium 6.20
pregnancy
   hormones 6.30
   hypertension 9.3

infections during 3.2, 3.10, 3.12
   teratogenic drugs 9.20
prevalence 8.13
prion diseases 3.14
prolactin 6.57
prospective (cohort) studies 8.6, 8.16
protein synthesis 2.17, 2.20
proteinuria 7.21
proto-oncogenes 2.4
pulmonary disease *see* lung

radial nerve 5.17
ras protein 2.19
rates, of disease 8.19
Raynaud's disease 6.17
   drug-induced 9.38
recreational drugs 9.49
reflexes 5.2
renal disease/physiology *see* kidney
renin
   release 6.31
   renin-angiotensin system 6.28
respiration *see* ventilation
respiratory disease *see* lung
retrospective (case-control) studies
   8.6, 8.16–17
rhesus factor 6.11
rheumatoid factor 4.7
RNA 2.20
rubella, congenital 3.10

sample size 8.14–15
screening tests 8.7, 8.10
senescence 2.21
sensitivity 8.7, 8.10
sex-linked inheritance 1.3–4
shock
   cardiogenic 5.30, 9.27
   hypovolaemic 6.4, 6.28
sickle cell disease 1.20, 3.9
sildenafil (Viagra®) 9.48
Sjögren's syndrome 1.5
skin
   innervation 5.10
   rashes 4.31
sodium 9.6
sodium valproate 9.44
specificity 8.7, 8.10

spinal cord   5.11, 5.27
  corticospinal pathway   5.25
  nerve roots   5.2, 5.10, 5.15, 5.21,
    5.28
  sensory pathways   6.36
standard deviation   8.2–3
standard error, of the mean (SEM)
  8.2
Staphylococcus aureus   3.18–19
  MRSA   3.38
Starling curve   6.5
steroids
  corticosteroids   6.9, 7.24
  in pregnancy   6.30
  receptors   2.14
stomach
  gastrin   6.39
  H. pylori   3.24
Streptococcus pneumoniae   3.22
stroke   5.24, 5.32
subclavian artery   5.1
sulphonylureas   9.8
sympathetic nervous system   6.17,
  6.38
systemic lupus erythematosus (SLE)
  4.24, 4.31

T cells   4.9
  antigen presentation   4.29–30
  CD antigens   4.33
  CD4/CD8 cells   4.5, 4.36
  helper T cells   4.27
tachycardia
  torsades de pointes   7.34
  Valsalva manoeuvre   6.1
tapeworms   7.12
teratogenic drugs   9.20
therapeutic drug monitoring   9.19
thiazides   9.45
thoracic duct   5.7
thyroid
  anatomy   5.19
  disease   6.57
torsades de pointes   7.34
toxoplasmosis   3.12, 3.29
transcription   2.17
transcription factors   2.14
transferrin   7.6

transforming growth factor-β (TGF-β)
  2.18
translation   2.17, 2.20
transmission of infectious diseases
  3.15, 3.33, 3.35
transplantation   4.1, 4.35
triglycerides   9.9
trinucleotide repeats   2.13
trochlear nerve   5.26
Trypanosoma brucei   4.25
tuberculosis
  M tuberculosis   3.17
  vaccination   4.15
tumour necrosis factor (TNF)   2.8,
  4.14
tumour suppressor genes   1.15, 2.5,
  2.9
Turner's syndrome   1.10, 1.13
type 1 error   8.14-15
type 2 error   8.15

ulnar nerve   5.5
upper limb   5.2, 5.5, 5.8–10, 5.17,
  5.21, 5.28
uric acid   7.32, 9.39
urine, discolouration   7.10

vaccination
  contraindications   3.11, 3.20,
    4.15
  hepatitis B   3.31
  S. pneumoniae   3.22
  TB   4.15
Valsalva manoeuvre   6.1
vasoactive intestinal peptide (VIP)
  6.14
vasoconstriction/dilatation   2.1,
  6.50
vasopressin (ADH)   6.18
vena cava, inferior   5.20
venous system, portosystemic
  anastomoses   5.12
ventilation
  control   6.7
  difficulties   6.10, 6.49
ventricles
  LVF   6.55
  outflow obstruction   6.54

Viagra® (sildenafil)   9.48
vincristine   9.43
viricides   3.32
vitamins
   B₁ 7.4
   B₁₂ 6.6, 7.12
   D   7.30
   K   6.15
vomiting   6.46
von Gierke's disease   7.1

warfarin   6.15
water balance   6.24, 6.42
Wegener's granulomatosis   4.19

Wernicke's encephalopathy   5.31,
   7.4
Wiskott–Aldrich syndrome   4.34
wrist   5.5

X-linked inheritance   1.3–4
xenotransplantation   4.35

yellow fever   3.5

zidovudine   9.10
zoonoses
   C. burnetii   3.36
   transmission   3.15, 3.33, 3.35

PasTest

PasTest has been established since 1972 and is the leading provider of exam-related medical revision course sand books in the UK. The company has a dedicated customer services team to ensure that doctors can easily get up to date information about our products and to ensure that their orders are dealt with efficiently. Our extensive experience means that we are always one step ahead when it comes to knowledge of the current trends and contents of the Royal College exams.

In the last 12 months we have sold over 67,000 books to medical students and qualified doctors. These may be purchased through bookshops, over the telephone or online at our website. All books are reviewed prior to publication to ensure that they mirror the needs of candidates and therefore act as an invaluable aid to exam preparation.

Test yourself online
PasTest Online is an extensive database of Best of Five questions written by experts to help you prepare for the MRCP Part 1 examination.

PasTest Online:

- enables you to test yourself whenever you want
- is accessible at any time
- is reasonably priced
- has a choice of mock exam, random questions and specialist questions. This means that you can test yourself in certain weak areas or take a mock exam.

Interested? Try a free demo at www.pastestonline.co.uk

100% Money Back Guarantee

We're sure you will find our study books invaluable, but in the unlikely event that you are not entirely happy, we will give you your money back – guaranteed.

Delivery to your Door

With a busy lifestyle, nobody enjoys walking to the shops for something that may or may not be in stock. Let us take the hassle and deliver direct to your door. We will despatch your book within 24 hours of receiving your order. We also offer free delivery on books for medical students to UK addresses.

How to Order

www.pastest.co.uk
To order books safely and securely online, shop at our website.

Telephone: +44 (0)1565 752000

Have your credit card to hand when you call.

+44 (0) 1565 650264

Fax your order with your debit or credit card details.

PasTest Ltd, FREEPOST, Knutsford, Cheshire WA16 7BR

Send your order with your cheque (made payable to PasTest Ltd) and debit or credit card details to the above address. (Please complete your address details on the reverse of the cheque.)